UNDERSTANDING
THE MENTALLY
RETARDED CHILD

Understanding the Mentally Retarded Child

A NEW APPROACH

by Richard Koch, M.D.,
and Kathryn Jean Koch

RANDOM HOUSE 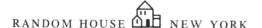 NEW YORK

Library of Congress Cataloging in Publication Data
Koch, Richard, 1921-
   Understanding the mentally retarded child.
   Bibliography: p.
   1. Mentally handicapped children. I. Koch, Kathryn Jean, joint author. II. Title. [DNLM: 1. Mental retardation—Popular works.   WS107 K76u]
RJ506.M4K57 1975   618.9′28′588   74-9087
ISBN 0-394-48547-5

ILLUSTRATIONS COURTESY OF DARREL DAVIS

Manufactured in the United States of America
9   8   7   6   5   4   3   2
First Edition

We dedicate this book,
our first joint literary effort,
to our other joint efforts:
Jill, Thomas, Christine, Martin and Leslie

Preface

It is indeed difficult for me to adequately express my praise for this desperately needed book from the medical field—bringing hope and promise for the retarded.

As the mother of a child who was born with Down's syndrome in August of 1950 and died two days before her second birthday, I can imagine the balm of tangible comfort and understanding this book will bring to those who happen to be part of the "three out of one hundred" whose children were born with abnormalities. My husband and I were two of those parents who were told: "Put her in an institution; she will never be normal; it isn't fair to your other children to take her home." Because of our Christian faith and the fact that we were very much in the public eye as entertainers at that time, we listened to the two doctors who said, "Take her home, love her, and do all you can for her as long as you have her."

The two years our little Robin lived taught us many wonderful lessons; our lives were enriched by her before God took her back to Himself. My husband and I did what we could for our child. At that time, medical science had little to offer in the way of tangible help, and I can well appreciate the keen hurt of the doctors who have to tell parents their newborn child is retarded and may never reach normalcy. When Robin was five weeks old, I read an article by the late Pearl Buck, entitled "My Child Stopped Growing." She said, "Never stop hoping—tomorrow there may be help for the retarded. It will probably be too late for my child, but maybe not for yours . . ."

This book has come too late for our child, but how I rejoice that others will be helped, the public further enlightened, and real light come into the lives of the "special ones" and their parents.

May God bless the writers and readers of this "oasis" book!

Dale Evans Rogers

Acknowledgments

Experience gained over the years has made possible the writing of this book. In addition, the encouragement and advice received from various friends and colleagues has been invaluable.

We wish to thank Betty Graliker, James Dobson, Lorraine Ogg, Karol Fishler, Philip Wiese, Ann Baerwald, Dolores Berkowitz, Kenneth Shaw and William Bucher. We also thank Evelyn Rabb and Tad Masaoka for the information they provided on citizenship and housing legislation; Elizabeth Wenz for donating material on the PKU diet; and our daughter, Chris, for writing the poetry for the book. A special thanks is due Mr. and Mrs. Marvin Pierce and Mr. and Mrs. Richard Kellis. We are indebted to

Michael Kaback for contributing from his broad background, as well as to William Green of the California Association for the Retarded; Philip Roos of the National Association for Retarded Citizens; and Robert Frazier of the American Academy of Pediatrics. Gratitude is also expressed to Dr. George Donnell, Henry Dunlap and Ronald Carson, the officials at the Childrens Hospital of Los Angeles for providing the facilities and opportunity to write this book.

Contents

Foreword

One of the pleasant duties of a physician is sharing in the joy of parents over the birth of a new baby. After the months of anticipation on the part of the family, there is nothing more enjoyable than to report, "You have a beautiful, healthy, normal new baby."

In three out of every hundred births, however, the doctor faces the difficult task of telling the parents that the child they have produced may never attain the mental capacities of a normal adult and that perhaps the child may also be physically handicapped. And the parents will have to adjust to the fact that the child they have wanted and planned for will always need extra care, help and understanding. Initially the parents may feel guilty about having produced such a child, or they may seek to blame each other. They will have a hundred questions. "Why did this happen to us?" "Is it hereditary?" "How long will he live?" "What will his future be?" The financial burden of raising such a child will place an added strain on their marital relationship. In their distress, they will need expert, sympathetic help and understanding.

Until a very few years ago, the medical profession was completely unprepared to deal with this all too common problem. The solution most commonly offered was, "Your child can never be normal. It's best to put it away in an institution and forget it was ever born." All infants suspected of being mentally retarded were lumped together into a sort of subhuman group—supposedly untreatable, untrainable—to be hidden away so that they could not harm others or offend the sensibilities of "normal" people.

Fortunately, today the medical profession and society as a whole are becoming more enlightened toward the problem of mental retardation. Much remains to be done, but progress is being made. It is now known that all forms of mental retardation are not the same. There are many degrees of retardation, ranging from the mild, or borderline, to the severe. Some of the causes are now known, and research is continuing in this field. In some cases, mental retardation can be cured or prevented. In fact, if all of the knowledge presently available to the medical profession were applied, the incidence of mental retardation in the United States could be cut in half. Experts are now able to diagnose and evaluate many of the disorders which cause mental retardation. There are individuals from many professions who are trained to help these children develop their fullest potential. Most professionals have realized that separating such children from their families and from society as a whole and locking them up in huge, isolated institutions is not the answer.

As those working in the field become more enlightened, parents of retarded children are being encouraged to keep their children in their homes whenever possible, or to place them in foster homes or small, homelike facilities when real home care is not possible. More and more, these children are seen with their families doing the things everyone enjoys—going to parks or to the beach, riding a bus to their job, or doing such chores as yard work. And more and more often, it is difficult to pick them out as they mingle with so-called normal people because, given the opportunity to develop, they are more normal than abnormal. They want to be useful and needed; they respond to friendliness and understanding. Above all, they want companionship, acceptance and love.

This book is written in the hope that it will help clarify the picture for the many families that are affected by the problem, and that it will help dispel the fear and apprehension with which the average person has viewed the mentally retarded in the past. Surely, in a mature society, all persons, regardless of the level of their intellectual ability, should and must be fully accepted.

Richard and Kathryn Jean Koch

UNDERSTANDING
THE MENTALLY
RETARDED CHILD

I

Mental Retardation, An Age-Old Problem

In earlier ages when only the fittest survived, those retarded children who also suffered from physical handicaps usually died young. Many primitive societies solved the problem by destroying any misshapen or obviously abnormal babies at birth. For example, in Hawaii, the abnormal newborn infant was placed at the water's edge to be engulfed by the incoming tide. And when the Roman emperor Vespasian captured opposing populations, all the infirm aged and handicapped were immediately put to death because the Romans wanted only prisoners who were able to work. Such barbaric practices were not limited to ancient times. As is well known, during the Nazi reign in Germany, many retarded persons were disposed of as if they were nonhuman.

There have been times when the retarded had preferential treatment. At one time it was fashionable in the courts of Europe to keep dwarfs as special pets and court jesters. Although some of them were undoubtedly retarded, they were thought to bring good luck.

During the early years of this nation, it is probable that some of the retarded were better off than they are today. The mildly retarded person in colonial America could perform farm work and household duties without having to contend with the competitiveness of today's science-oriented society. In some cases, there were enough maiden aunts or other brothers and sisters in the home, so that the child fared not too badly. And no doubt, in the South, before the Civil War, the task of overseeing a retarded child was assigned to a servant or slave.

But more often since the beginning of time, the lot of the retarded has been a painful one. There have always been the cases of children being hidden away, living out their lives tied up in some attic or basement because of the embarrassment the family would suffer if the child were discovered. Such cases still occasionally come to light.

During the Middle Ages, throughout Europe, ignorance and superstition combined with the overzealousness of church officials and civil judges to produce a mass hysteria which resulted in thousands of people being tortured and put to death as witches or warlocks. Churchmen were particularly vengeful in their efforts to kill all witches. Did not the Bible (Exodus 22:18) command them, "Thou shalt not suffer a witch to live"? In the light of modern knowledge, it seems obvious that many of the people who were considered to be under the spell of witches or possessed by the devil were actually mentally ill or retarded. Witchcraft trial records state in detail the symptoms of people under the spell of witches; some of the descriptions are clear pictures of people suffering epileptic seizures. Nor was this country free from the mass madness of witch hunts. We will probably never know how many retarded persons were put to death by our Puritan forefathers as witches. One thing we do know; anyone appearing or acting a little "different" came under suspicion.

The advent of "hospitals" and asylums for the mentally incompetent coincided with the cessation of witch hunting. The first hospital for the mentally ill in the United States was built in Williamsburg, Virginia, in 1773. These asylums were more like prisons than hospitals, where the poor victims were chained in tiny cells without heat or proper food. And some of the medical treatments used to try to cure them were little better than the tortures used to gain confessions from witches in earlier years.

In this century, the so-called intelligence quotient (IQ) is used to measure the mental capacity of individuals. The highest score is 200; scores in the lower range between 0 and 70 indicate mental retardation. But mental retardation is more than a score on a test. The American Association for Mental Deficiency defines mental retardation as "subaverage general intellectual functioning which originates during the developmental period (conception to seventeen years) and is associated with impairment in adaptive behavior." In other words, the mentally retarded person is one who has suffered an impairment of his ability to think, learn and reason. The cause of this impairment may have occurred at the time he was conceived, during the period of gestation, during the birth process, or during his infancy or childhood. The cause may be known, but more often it is not. It may be a hereditary condition, or it may merely be an unfortunate accident of nature. While mental retardation can occur in a wide range of severity, it is nearly always a chronic disorder which cannot be cured in the usual sense, but whose effects can often be minimized.

Until a very few years ago, the first-grader who could

not learn to read, or who printed his letters backward or upside down, or who may have been clumsy on the playground was soon looked upon as a dummy by his classmates. He was ostracized from their games and parties. If he was lucky, he had understanding parents and a teacher knowledgeable about such problems. But all too often, the adults with whom he had to interact were too preoccupied with other problems, or were so imperceptive that they merely added to the difficulty.

As such a child grew older, he often turned to antisocial behavior to gain the recognition he could not gain through scholastic or athletic achievement. If this cycle of rejection by society followed by antisocial behavior continued long enough, the individual eventually ended up as a complete liability, locked up in a prison or some sort of institution. It is a fact that some of the men who have been executed in our prisons have been retarded. Statistics are difficult to obtain, but we have been able to examine a study made by Robert M. Carter in 1953 of those men who were executed in California between 1938 and 1953. No intelligence level was available in some cases, but of those on whom this information was available, 45 percent were in the borderline-defective to dull-normal range. And as late as 1959–1962, of those on whom intelligence levels were available, 14.8 percent were in this same low range. We feel that this indicates not that the mentally retarded usually have criminal-type personalities, but that society has turned its back for too long on the problems of the retarded. For too long, the personalities of retarded children have been warped by the cruel ostracism of their classmates and the lack of understanding of parents and other adults. Only when they finally committed a crime did society give attention by seeking punishment and retribution.

Even today many mentally retarded persons are in our

penal and mental institutions. Our society has placed great importance on conforming to its standards, and those individuals who, for some reason, do not or cannot conform learn that they are not accepted by society. If they choose an unusual hair or dress style, they may be unable to secure employment; if they choose some unusual life style, they may find themselves ostracized by their more conformist neighbors. How much worse, then, is the lot of the retarded, who cannot help being different. In some cases, they have unusual facial features; they may have awkward speech patterns and strange mannerisms. We no longer put them to death or lock them up in attics, but until very recently, modern society has reacted by isolating them in large institutions where they are invisible to the general public. Even as late as 1953, one well-known medical textbook said of the retarded, "Institutional training is the best available form of treatment." It has only been within the past ten years that the medical profession has really accepted responsibility for dealing with the retarded.

It is obvious that throughout history the retarded have been the victims of circumstance. They have been an embarrassment to their families and a thorn in the flesh of society. Despite the progress that has been made, disclosures in New York and Arkansas as recently as 1972 have shown us that many of our modern institutions for the retarded are no better than were the snake pits of a hundred years ago.

Before the development of antibiotics, doctors did well to care for routine infectious diseases. Even since the medical profession has been able to cure most infections, how much more gratifying it is for a doctor to treat a child with an infected ear which can be cured by penicillin than to deal with the medical problems of a child with an IQ of 50. How much more pleasant for a surgeon to remove an infected appendix than to correct a physical handicap in a retarded child.

Teachers were the first professional group to realize their responsibility toward the retarded. The classroom teacher was often the first to suspect mental retardation in a child who had special problems with academic subjects. But it was not until the 1950's that special education courses were offered to teachers interested in working with educationally handicapped children. In most states it is now mandatory for the public schools to have programs for educable and trainable children, and a few states have new laws providing special education for every physically and mentally handicapped child, no matter how seriously disabled. Teachers now provide 75 percent of the services to the mentally retarded.

Other professions have slowly come to realize that they, too, have a responsibility toward the retarded and their families. They are represented in a broad range that includes psychologists, hearing and speech experts, nutritionists, social workers, nurses and biochemists.

The parents with a retarded child need no longer feel that they must struggle alone with insurmountable problems. They may turn to professionals in the field and to a number of voluntary organizations, such as the National Association for Retarded Citizens (formerly the National Association for Retarded Children), which has chapters in many cities throughout the country.

In our society we have learned to accept and work with persons with physical defects; the birth of a child with clubfeet or a harelip and cleft palate is no longer the tragedy it once was. Now we are approaching a new maturity in which a mentally retarded child is viewed as a person with the same right as others to develop his highest potential. The turning point in the attitude toward mental retardation in this country began in 1950 with the establishment of the National Association for Retarded Children, an organization of parents working for the welfare of their retarded family members. In 1973 the name of the organization was changed to National Association for Retarded Citizens because the members felt a responsibility for helping retarded people, regardless of their age. Much of the real progress occurred in the 1960's when President John Kennedy, who had a retarded sister, focused attention on the problem by establishing the President's Panel on Mental Retardation, a 21-member group of outstanding professionals and laymen in the field who studied the overall problem in this country and abroad. The group prepared an extensive report, much of which has been implemented by legislation benefiting the retarded.

The early progress of the fifties and sixties gathered momentum, and in 1968 the Assembly of the International League of Societies for the Mentally Handicapped adopted the following declaration of the general and special rights of the mentally retarded.

Whereas the universal declaration of human rights, adopted by the United Nations proclaims that all of the human family, without distinction of any kind, have equal and inalienable rights of human dignity and freedom;

Whereas the declaration of the rights of the child, adopted by the United Nations, proclaims the rights of the physically, mentally or socially handicapped child to special treatment, education and care required by his particular condition.

NOW THEREFORE

The International League of Societies for the Mentally Handicapped expresses the general and special rights of the mentally retarded as follows:

Article I

The mentally retarded person has the same basic rights as other citizens of the same country and same age.

Article II

The mentally retarded person has a right to proper medical care and physical restoration and to such education, training, habilitation and guidance as will enable him to develop his ability and potential to the fullest possible extent, no matter how severe his degree of disability. No mentally handicapped person should be deprived of such services by reason of the costs involved.

Article III

The mentally retarded person has a right to economic security and to a decent standard of living. He has a right to productive work or to other meaningful occupation.

Article IV

The mentally retarded person has a right to live with his own family or with foster parents: to participate in all aspects of community life, and to be provided with appropriate leisure-time activities. If care in an institution becomes necessary, it should be in surroundings and under circumstances as close to normal living as possible.

Article V

The mentally retarded person has a right to a qualified guardian when this is required to protect his personal well-being and interest. No person rendering direct services to the mentally retarded should also serve as his guardian.

Article VI

The mentally retarded person has a right to protection from exploitation, abuse and degrading treatment. If accused, he has a right to a fair trial with full recognition being given to his degree of responsibility.

Article VII

Some mentally retarded persons may be unable, due to the severity of their handicap, to exercise for themselves all of their rights in a meaningful way. For others, modification of some or all of these rights is appropriate. The procedure used for modification or denial of rights must contain proper legal safeguards against every form of abuse, must be based on an evaluation of the social capability of the mentally retarded person by qualified experts and must be subject to periodic reviews and to the right of appeal to higher authorities. ABOVE ALL— THE MENTALLY RETARDED PERSON HAS THE RIGHT TO RESPECT.

III

What Is Mental Retardation?

When the doctor reports, "Your child is mentally retarded," what does he mean? It must first be understood that mental retardation is not a specific disorder in itself but a symptom associated with a number of disorders. In some cases, it occurs in association with physical handicaps or an unusual appearance. When mental retardation is accompanied by other symptoms which all point to a specific condition, the disorder is called a syndrome.

There are many syndromes known to medical science which are associated with mental retardation, in which the individuals bear a set of distinguishing characteristics. The most common example is Down's syndrome, a chromosome disorder which will be discussed in detail in a later chapter.

It is sufficient to note here that individuals with Down's syndrome (or Mongolism, as it was formerly called) have certain features in common. They have eyes that look Oriental; they are short in stature and often heavy; they have stubby hands and feet; and they are usually mentally retarded. In Down's syndrome, and in nearly all disorders causing mental retardation, there is a wide range of severity. Given the proper training and opportunity, many of the borderline or mildly retarded people are able to fit into the normal population, and become useful, active members of society. This is why it was so unjust that all retarded individuals were labeled as hopeless, separated from their families, and denied all forms of stimulation and training during infancy. Locked away in institutions, it was no wonder that they truly deteriorated into hopeless retardation.

How are the retarded different from the general population? As infants, they are usually slow in developing. They do not smile at the age of two to six weeks, as do normal infants. Their sitting up, crawling and walking are delayed. Speech is also slow in developing, and, of course, in severe retardation, the patient never learns to talk. According to studies done by Arnold Gesell of Yale University, in which a large number of babies were observed, the following pattern of development should be considered normal:

> *1 month:* Begins to have some regard of his surroundings.
>
> *2 months:* Begins to smile and vocalizes by cooing.
>
> *3 months:* Has head control and turns in the direction of sound.

4 months:	Reaches to grasp objects with both hands.
5 months:	Rolls over.
6 months:	Begins to transfer objects from hand to hand.
7 months:	Sits alone.
8 months:	Creeps.
9 months:	Pulls up and begins to use forefinger-thumb opposition.
10 months:	Stands, holding on.
12 months:	Stands alone and begins to use single words.
12-15 months:	Walks alone and creeps upstairs.
15-18 months:	Walks and rarely falls; begins to throw a ball.
18-24 months:	Runs, climbs, jumps, walks upstairs, kicks a ball, points to various parts of the body, puts two words together.

These milestones are averages; not all children will achieve them as early as the average, and some will be ahead of schedule. They are merely the norm for purposes of comparison. Most retarded children will fall far behind in many of the categories. There are some children, however, who lag considerably behind this pattern of achievements who are not mentally retarded. They suffer from some other disorder, such as a severe hearing loss, which prevents them from developing at the same rate as other children who have no handicap. These children are said to be pseudo-retarded. (Pseudo-retardation will be discussed in more detail in a later chapter.) Mental retardation is often associated with seizures (temporary loss of consciousness). It can also be associated with cerebral palsy, in which there is a lack of muscular coordination, and with abnormalities of head size and shape (the head may be either extremely large or small).

Mental retardation is not always recognizable at birth. In some mild cases it does not become obvious until the child enters school and is unable to learn to read and write.

Until about the middle of this century, professionals indicated the degree of retardation by such terms as idiot, imbecile, moron or dull-witted. The retarded are no longer classified in this way. In England and some other countries, the terms "backward" or "subnormal" are used. Through psychological testing and observation, it is possible for psychologists to make some determination of the IQ level at which a child is functioning. In general, professionals consider individuals with nonmeasurable IQ's to be profoundly retarded; an IQ between 1 and 29 indicates severe retardation. Four percent of retarded persons are in the profoundly and severely retarded range. These individuals are usually not toilet-trained and generally have severe health problems requiring skilled nursing care. They are nearly always completely dependent; these are the persons who may eventually need care outside their own homes, since few families are able to provide the 24-hour-a-day supervision and care necessary for such an individual. Their life span is usually only twenty to twenty-five years because of their many health problems.

A person with an IQ between 30 and 50 is considered to be moderately retarded. Twenty-one percent of the retarded fall into this category. The moderately retarded can learn simple speech, but they need supervision all of their lives. They are considered to be trainable, which means that they can be toilet-trained and taught to dress and feed themselves. If properly trained, they can learn simple tasks so that they can work in sheltered workshops. These workshops afford such a person the protection and guidance he needs, as they are usually supervised by specialists. The employee also gains self-respect and a feeling of usefulness because he is paid a salary for producing a product or performing a service. These workshops can be found in most major cities in the United States and abroad. The local chapters of the National Association for Retarded Citizens have information on sheltered workshops in their areas. Their work varies from simple crafts, such as candle-making and rug weaving to the assembly of complicated electronics equipment. They sometimes have contracts to package certain products for mailing. One workshop in California packages the earphone sets used by airline passengers for music and movies while in flight. The work produced in a sheltered workshop depends to a great degree upon the resourcefulness and ingenuity of its director in devising simple, easily understood instructions and assembly techniques as well as the willingness of companies within the community to give contracts to the workshop.

The description of the above categories of mental retardation may be useful as a guide to parents and professionals, but there are individuals who do not fit neatly into these classifications. For example, the multiply-handicapped person who cannot walk because of lack of muscle control, is unable to feed himself or become toilet-trained may have normal intelligence. Also, some totally deaf persons never learn to talk, but have normal intelligence.

While the different categories of mental retardation are classified according to IQ level, it should be emphasized that these categories have been established in order to facilitate the work of professionals in this field. For example, a school psychologist finding that a child has an IQ of 40 would send the child to a class for the trainable mentally retarded, since an IQ between 30 and 50 indicates trainable mental retardation. The child with an IQ between 50 and

70 would be sent to a class for the educable mentally retarded. The classification has provided access into a school program for the child.

While there are advantages to such classifications, there are also disadvantages. There is always the danger of labeling a person as belonging to a certain classification, regardless of his actual level of functioning. In fact, until recent years, the IQ was thought to be an unchanging figure; once a person was labeled as mentally retarded, it was thought he would always be mentally retarded. Professionals have now realized the fallacy of this theory, and it is one we should all guard against. Intelligence quotient is not static: it can become higher or lower, depending upon many factors. Special-education teachers are alert to the fact that children must be placed in the proper program. If a child in a class for the trainable retarded is found to be functioning at a more advanced level, he is transferred to a class for the educable retarded. Sometimes children in classes for the educable retarded are able to go into regular school classes; conversely, sometimes children who are having a difficult struggle in regular classes are helped by going into classes for the educable retarded.

As the mentally retarded become accepted in school programs and in the community, it is increasingly evident that there are many more facets to personality and intelligence than the IQ. Some children who cannot go beyond third-grade arithmetic have great artistic talent. Their talent should be cultivated and they should feel pride in their artistic achievements. Other retarded people write poetry. Some girls who are mildly retarded in schools marry and become very good homemakers and mothers. Often moderately and even severely retarded people have remarkable musical ability. The authors have seen a child who was unable to read music learn to play complicated piano compositions. His innovative teacher realized his potential and was willing to experiment. The boy was taught by having his fingers taped to the teacher's fingers. As she played the music, he was able to memorize the positions and patterns of the fingering; after a few weeks of practicing in this manner, the tapes were removed, and he was able to play the music. As a result of this achievement, his interest grew and he is now learning to read music. This has opened a whole new outlet for him, and his pride in his accomplishments has changed his whole personality.

Of special importance is the fact that after the average person finishes school, purely intellectual achievements are not really so important. Of equal or more importance are such character traits as a pleasant personality, honesty and thoughtfulness. We have all known some very intelligent people who are constantly unhappy and who communicate this unhappiness by being unpleasant to everyone around them. It is doubtful that anyone would prefer the company of a chronic complainer, just because he had a high IQ, to that of someone else who, though not particularly intellectual, has a happy, uncomplaining personality.

This being so, we would offer this advice to the parents of retarded children. Remember that your child's IQ level is not as important as his ability to be socially acceptable. People will not really be impressed with the fact that he learned to read at the age of three or the age of thirteen if he goes about spitting on people or drawing pictures on the walls. A child in a class for the educable retarded should eventually be qualified to earn his own living, but he may be unable to do so if he is constantly hitting people to get attention; in contrast to this, a well-behaved person with an IQ of only 50 may be able to become independent. Although the retarded child may not intuitively sense what is socially acceptable, as most normal children do, he can be taught. Through patience and persistence and love, parents can teach a retarded child to be well-mannered and pleasant—a person people like to be with. For any parent, this is an accomplishment to be proud of.

IIII

Conquering Mental Retardation through Programs of Prevention

The most exciting aspect of the field of mental retardation is the relatively new area of prevention. In the past, the discoveries of vaccines against diseases such as smallpox, diphtheria and whooping cough have been applauded. More recently, we have seen the development of the poliomyelitis vaccine. Some of the recent advances in techniques for preventing mental retardation will have a dramatic impact on the whole field of preventive medicine. As a matter of fact, even now the tools are available to the medical profession to cut the incidence of mental retardation by 50 percent. What is deplorable is that we have not taken full advantage of these procedures.

It is now well known that babies whose mothers have

had German measles (rubella) during the first three months of pregnancy are nearly always born with multiple defects, including mental retardation. However, it is not well known that since 1970 there has been a vaccine that can give lifetime protection against this disease. The vaccine, which is composed of attenuated (weakened) rubella viruses, normally causes no adverse reaction when it is administered, but it does cause the system to produce rubella antibodies. It is no longer necessary for any woman to run the risk of contracting German measles during her pregnancy. Little has been done, however, to publicize this important development. On the contrary, the members of the California Medical Association, on the advice of the Public Health Service, have been adamant in refusing to administer this vaccine to any girl over the age of thirteen years. The reason for this seemingly incongruous decision is the fear of malpractice suits on the part of most doctors. Their reasoning is that since the vaccine causes the woman's system to produce rubella antibodies, it might cause damage to a fetus if it is administered to a pregnant woman—and any girl thirteen years old has presumably reached puberty and therefore might be pregnant! Recent evidence suggests that this fear is ungrounded. A number of women who did not know they were pregnant were immunized against rubella. When it was discovered that they had been pregnant at the time of immunization, they were given the opportunity to have therapeutic abortions, and some of them elected to do so, rather than run the risk of producing a defective child. Upon examination of the aborted fetuses, it was found that none showed any effects of the virus. And among those who did not have abortions, all but one of the infants were normal. All a doctor need do is to test a sample of a girl's blood for antibodies against German measles to determine for sure whether or not she has had the disease. If no antibodies are found, she has never had German measles, and should be vaccinated against it. If the doctor has any doubts as to whether or not the patient is pregnant, a pregnancy test will rule out this complication before the vaccine is given.

There is at least one case in which a woman who was denied the vaccine subsequently became pregnant, contracted German measles during the pregnancy, and gave birth to an abnormal child. She has brought suit for malpractice against the doctor who refused her the inoculation. This case may provide a precedent, so that physicians will take a more realistic approach to this problem in the future. According to the President's Committee on Mental Retardation, 10 to 25 percent of all women of child-bearing age are considered to be at risk in terms of contracting rubella; in other words, they are susceptible to German measles and could catch it if exposed. *Every girl who has not had German measles by her twelfth year should be given the vaccine.*

The California Legislature recently passed a bill requiring that the premarital blood sample on women be tested for rubella as well as syphilis antibodies. The importance of the vaccination is explained to them and they are urged to go to the local health department or to their private physicians for an immunization if no rubella antibodies are found. This law went into effect on January 1, 1974. Although such legislation as this helps to make people aware of the problem, more public education is urgently needed in this area.

Another way in which mental retardation can be prevented is to make sure that the population is protected against the other common diseases for which we have vaccines, because complications from these diseases can cause mental retardation. Why is it that even today, our population is not totally protected against measles, poliomyelitis, diphtheria, tetanus and whooping cough? Adequate amounts of vaccine are available, and certainly manpower is sufficient. It seems that our national priorities have been misplaced. Is it the system of providing medical care that is at fault or is it the inherent lethargy of people? Perhaps too many people are unaware of the untold tragedies which result from unnecessary illness. In any case, it is inexcusable that the medical profession has not done more to educate the public on the importance of preventive measures.

There are other changes that are urgently needed if we are to prevent the occurrence of mental retardation. It may take an aroused citizenry to bring about these changes, since much of the time the medical profession seems to be crisis-oriented. Mental retardation is neither a crisis, nor is it dramatic. But it is a field in which exciting progress can be made if the necessary changes are instituted.

There are some exemplary programs throughout our country today. For example, Massachusetts has a testing program in which all newborn babies are given blood and urine tests to detect twenty to thirty different inherited diseases which cause mental retardation. This is the most complete testing program being carried out in the United States. Of course, some of these diseases are, as yet, untreatable, but genetic counseling in such cases helps the parents as they weigh the pros and cons of having other children, and in most of these cases they decide against having other children of their own. Seven of the diseases can be effectively treated by special diets and mental retardation prevented. Imagine the suffering and hardship that could be prevented if each state had such a program.

Some states have made notable progress in the management of premature infants by developing special centers where all such infants are taken immediately after birth. In these modern centers the latest techniques are used in an effort to help the tiny babies develop normally. There are nurses who are specially trained in working with premature babies. Special formulas are available for infants with feeding problems. There are special oxygen-measuring instruments which regulate the flow of oxygen to the babies, so that their eyes are not damaged by an excess amount. In former years many premature infants suffered blindness as a result of the fact that their oxygen supply was not measured. New York and a few other states have these programs for premature infants. We should have them in all states.

On January 1, 1974, California instituted a new program to do mass screening of all Jewish men and women to detect the carriers of Tay-Sachs Disease, a devastating hereditary disorder which strikes one out of every 3,600 infants whose parents are descended from Ashkenazi Jews. The disease is always fatal, with the infant deteriorating progressively and becoming blind and mentally retarded. The children usually live three to five years. A test which is 100 percent accurate in detecting the carriers of this disorder was developed in 1969. It is only when two carriers marry that the offspring will suffer from the disease; for such a couple, one out of four of their children will be a victim of Tay-Sachs Disease, two out of four will be carriers, and only one will be completely normal. Those persons who are found to be carriers of the disorder receive appropriate genetic counseling. California alone has a half million Jews who can be helped by this program. Such a program conducted on a nation-wide basis could be very effective in eradicating this disease.

It is important for everyone to realize that premature birth is a cause of mental retardation, and that the premature birth rate is related to economic factors. Each year there are about 330,000 premature babies, or 8 percent of all live births. The rate of prematurity is two to three times higher among women who have had little or no prenatal care, and the rate of prematurity in poverty areas is four to five times that in our well-to-do suburban areas. Since prematurity is directly related to the problem of mental retardation, we must make every effort to reduce it to the lowest possible figure. How incongruous it is that society is willing to pay for thirty years' care in an institution at $10,000 a year for each retarded person, but is unwilling to pay for the comparatively small cost of good prenatal care to prevent the mental retardation!

Perhaps the public schools should share in the responsibility of spreading vital information. Sex education and health classes could be combined into family relations classes encompassing not only sex education and health but preventive medicine and drug education. Such a program might take away the stigma of the title "sex education," which has become a scare term to many people, and provide the students with a well-rounded fund of information which could be invaluable to them in later life.

In 1966, routine testing of all newborn infants for phenylketonuria (PKU), a treatable disorder, was instituted in California. Subsequently forty-three other states have set up mass testing programs for PKU. These programs are called population screening, and they are becoming increasingly important. In the case of PKU, if the victims are not treated they almost invariably become severely mentally retarded. For PKU screening, all the newborns are given a blood test to detect the disorder before they leave the hospital. PKU is a hereditary disease in which the body is unable to properly use certain protein substances which are in many foods. These substances build up in the infant's system and cause brain damage, usually before the first year. Although there is no cure for PKU, there is a special diet which eliminates the harmful proteins. If the disease is diagnosed and the diet instituted early in infancy, mental retardation can be prevented.

Although pediatricians for years have been advocating routine physical examinations for newborns, they have felt uncomfortable about routine biochemical screening techniques. One famous, venerable pediatrician, when asked about routine screening, snorted his disgust at the idea by saying to his students, "We are trying to teach you to be clinicians and not to be dependent upon any laboratory test." Noble as this concept might have been twenty years ago (when a blood count, tuberculin skin test and a blood test for syphilis were the only routine laboratory studies performed), any pediatrician would be negligent today if he did not routinely test his patients for a variety of disorders which can be detected by blood and urine tests. Some twenty to thirty diseases which cause mental retardation can now be detected by these screening tests. The importance of these tests becomes obvious when one realizes that infants with these insidious diseases, which cause gradual degeneration, appear normal at birth. If such a disorder is not diagnosed until symptoms appear, brain damage has already occurred and it is too late to remedy the situation.

Galactosemia, histidinemia, homocystinuria, methylmalonicaciduria, hyperglycinemia and maple syrup urine disease are all hereditary disorders causing mental retardation which can be detected by screening tests. They are all characterized by progressive physical and mental degeneration. The patients may develop seizures; few of them ever learn to walk and talk, and they become severely retarded. Now, however, there are treatments for all of these diseases, so that mental retardation can usually be prevented if they are diagnosed before brain damage occurs.

Unfortunately, treatments have not been developed for all of the diseases which can be detected through screening. Niemann-Pick's Disease and Hurler's Disease are all hereditary disorders which cause progressive physical and mental retardation, and their victims usually do not live long. The advantage of diagnosing these diseases is that couples who have had a child afflicted with one of these disorders would know the risk involved in having another. They would be counseled against having other children of their own, and adoption would be suggested as an alternative if they wished to have other children. With amniocentesis a new approach is available.

One cause of mental retardation which is difficult to control and even more difficult to understand is child beating. Children who are beaten often suffer permanent brain damage because of repeated blows on the head. Efforts are currently being made to deal more effectively with this problem. There are sixty thousand cases of child abuse in the United States each year, and it is estimated that there are thousands of cases which go unreported. Professionals working in this field have found that child abusers are found at every economic level.

A self-help organization called Parents Anonymous was founded in Redondo Beach, California, in 1971. It now has a membership of four thousand confessed child abusers. Many of them were abused themselves as children, and they are often lonely, unhappy people. Usually in cases of child beating, the marriage is unstable, and the partners are often young, or there may be only one parent in the family. Sometimes, the father subconsciously wants the baby out of the way because it is taking too much of the mother's attention. Or in some cases, the mother may become distraught when the baby is especially irritable. They are usually truly sorry and are very solicitous after the child is injured. Dr. C. Henry Kempe, director of the National Center for Prevention of Child Abuse and Neglect, says that 90 percent of the child abusers can be cured and that only 10 percent are truly psychopathic individuals who should be permanently separated from their children.

Dr. Kempe's center in Denver, Colorado, was founded in 1972. Dr. Kempe feels that jailing child abusers is not the right solution, since imprisonment does not solve their basic problem. At his center, a team approach is used in dealing with these people. The team, made up of a pediatrician, social worker, police representative, psychiatrist and nurse, makes a complete evaluation of the parents and the child. A temporary guardian is named, and the team usually recommends foster care for the child while the parents are under treatment. The center uses the services of lay therapists, who need not have any particular formal education but must be dedicated and available night or day in a crisis. They are assigned to befriend parents who have beaten their child. They are paid two dollars an hour. The parents attend Families Anonymous, a group similar to Parents Anonymous, which holds weekly meetings so that they may talk with other parents about their mutual problems. Each parent is on call to help another when a crisis arises. There are also day-care facilities where parents can leave their child on a regular basis for a few hours at a time to give them some relief from the constant care required by a small child. The team determines when it is safe to let a child go home to his parents. In 10 percent of the cases, the child is allowed to return home within eight months. In four years of using the team approach to the problem, and of supplementing it with the services now consolidated at the center, Dr. Kempe has dealt with one thousand child-abuse cases, and has yet to see an instance in which beating has occurred after treatment. Similar programs in every major medical center would go far toward eliminating the problem of the battered child, but unfortunately, not all authorities are as forward-looking as Dr. Kempe.

Glandular disorders, such as hypothyroidism, are another preventable cause of mental retardation. At Pacific State Hospital for the retarded in Pomona, California, 1 percent of the residents are there because of hypothyroidism. If this disorder is diagnosed before brain damage occurs, mental retardation can be prevented through treatment with thyroid extract. Medical science now has a technique for detecting hypothyroidism when an infant is two months of age. However, the test is complicated and expensive. We hope that technology will soon make it possible to identify hypothyroid function by developing a simple, inexpensive test which could be administered to all two-month-old infants.

Although there has been increased publicity in recent years regarding the danger of cigarette smoking, most women do not realize that they can harm their unborn child by excessive smoking during pregnancy. This fact has been proven in a number of studies. The most significant was done by the Institute of Neurological Diseases and Blindness. It was found in a study of 40,000 pregnancies that there was a definite relationship between the number of cigarettes smoked by the mother and birth weight of her baby. The more cigarettes she smoked, the smaller was the baby at birth. It is an established fact that the smaller and more immature a baby is, the greater is the chance that it will not develop normally.

Mothers with severe diabetes and other chronic diseases should be counseled against having babies of their own since the occurrence of defects is greater in a mother with any chronic disease.

Every prospective mother should be made aware of the importance of knowing whether she and her husband are Rh compatible. The Rh factor refers to a normal condition of the blood cells. Everyone is either Rh positive or Rh negative. If both parents are Rh positive, or if they are both Rh negative, or if the father is Rh negative and the mother Rh positive, their children are unaffected. However, in the rare cases when the mother is Rh negative and the father Rh positive, the mother's body develops antibodies to the Rh factor in the unborn infant's blood. Fortunately, the first-born child of such a couple is not affected unless the mother has had a blood transfusion at some time during her life which has stimulated the production of the antibodies. However, subsequent children can be damaged and suffer mental retardation due to the destruction of fetal blood cells by the antibodies of the mother's system. Until recent years, an infant who suffered from this condition had to have a complete exchange of blood soon after birth, but today the mother can have an immunization which prevents her body from producing antibodies against the Rh factor and thus completely removes the risk from the pregnancy. The name of the immunizing product is Rhogam.

Another step in the prevention of mental retardation is better maternity care. The changes in our welfare system allowing lower-income families to utilize community services and private-practice facilities have been a significant step forward. The development of the maternity nurse-practitioner in prenatal care is another aspect of improved maternity care. This new professional provides prenatal care in uncomplicated cases, leaving the obstetrician more time to give to the complicated cases which need special expertise. This program, which has operated for some time in the hills of Kentucky and Tennessee has now been adopted by some areas of California. The widespread use of this program would be very effective in providing good prenatal care on a national basis. Better maternity care would reduce the possibility of complications resulting from conditions such as toxemia of pregnancy, placenta previa and traumatic birth.

Toxemia is developed by some women during the last three months of pregnancy. The causes are unknown, but the symptoms are high blood pressure, albumin in the urine, dizzy spells and, in severe cases, convulsions. If the patient is put on a low salt diet and given medication for the high blood pressure, the symptoms are usually controlled. If it is untreated the child is often born prematurely, with an increased risk of mental retardation.

In placenta previa, the placenta separates from the uterine wall during the birth process. Since the placenta supplies food and oxygen to the fetus during the pregnancy and birth process, it must remain attached to the uterine wall until the baby breathes by itself; otherwise the infant will suffer brain damage due to lack of oxygen. The experienced obstetrician can detect placenta previa before the onset of labor and deliver the baby by Caesarean operation, eliminating the chances of anoxia in the infant.

A traumatic birth refers to any complication which can occur during delivery, such as a breech or transverse position of the baby, or a very rapid or very long labor. These complications all require the skill of an experienced obstetrician.

In 1973 the United States Supreme Court upheld the legality of abortion during the first three months of pregnancy. Obstetricians are less busy with prenatal care and delivery and can provide better services to the populace as a whole. They can be invaluable as members of genetic counseling teams. They can also establish outreach programs in poverty areas. For example, if a prenatal clinic were held one evening a week in a minority community, the women would not have to take time off from work to go to the county hospital and wait in line for a checkup. Such an innovation would probably cut down significantly on the number of women having no prenatal care.

Probably the most exciting advancement in the field of prevention of mental retardation has been the development of a technique called amniocentesis. This is a diagnostic procedure which permits doctors to detect a number of diseases which cause severe mental retardation in utero (in the uterus) during the third month of pregnancy. In this test, a needle is inserted through the abdominal wall and into the uterus, and some of the amniotic fluid which surrounds the fetus is withdrawn. This fluid contains enough free-floating cells from the fetus to provide an adequate sample that can be examined in the laboratory for abnormalities. For example, the fetus with Down's syndrome can be identified, since it is now known that persons with Down's syndrome always have an extra chromosome in each cell. Through a technique called cytogenetics, the chromosomes can now be counted in the laboratory. The amniotic fluid can also be tested for Tay-Sachs Disease.

In addition, German measles and cytomegalo virus can be detected by amniocentesis. The results of maternal German measles are well known. Cytomegalo virus also affects the unborn infant, causing seizures and mental retardation.

With the perfecting of this technique of amniocentesis by obstetricians, it is being used increasingly in cases where there is a suspicion that a fetus may be developing abnormally. These recent advancements, along with the development of reliable contraceptives and the Supreme Court decision on abortions, have given new impetus to the field of genetic counseling.

Although genetic counseling is thought of as a modern science, it actually has been practiced for hundreds of years. Going back to the twelfth and thirteenth centuries, the Talmud of the Jews specified that a person could not marry if epilepsy had occurred within his family during the past two generations. It is no longer necessary to say that carriers of a genetic defect should not marry. The tools are now at hand to prevent the conception of infants with many types of handicaps. And in many cases, even after a potentially handicapped infant has been conceived, the medical and legal community can now safely terminate the pregnancy.

This decision to end a pregnancy is now, as it should be, the responsibility of the family involved and their physician. Abortion must no longer be cloaked in religiosity. The myths surrounding this subject must be put to rest. It has been postulated that abortion can cause psychological damage and depression in a woman. It is our firm belief that a woman is much more likely to suffer psychological damage and depression if she knows she is carrying a defective child but is prevented from terminating the pregnancy.

A word should be said here about those women whose religion prohibits contraception and abortion. The Catholic Church has always been at the forefront in opposing all mechanical and chemical forms of birth control, and in teaching that abortion is not to be condoned under any circumstances. In recent years, there has been a divergence of opinion among Catholic theologians regarding the use of contraceptives, and at present there is a trend among the Catholic clergy to "keep out of the bedroom." Many conscientious Catholic women are using the pill without opposition from their priests. This trend probably began when the Second Vatican Council, a body of 2,700 members, said that conscience is a guiding principle parallel to ecclesiastical authority in the life of a Christian. Although Pope Paul VI subsequently condemned all mechanical and chemical forms of birth control, many conscientious Catholics and concerned clergymen feel that the Pope's encyclical *Humanae Vitae* is merely a firm suggestion of how a Catholic should behave, rather than an absolute condemnation of contraceptives.

Increasingly, the Church is emphasizing the importance of family planning, and family-planning counseling is available at Catholic social service agencies. Of special interest is the teaching of the Church that a woman with a pathological condition which causes her to bear defective children should not bear children of her own. At the present time there is a movement among Catholic theologians to apply this principle to couples who run a high risk of producing abnormal children.

In a case where both partners carry a recessive genetic defect, making it probable that one in four of their children will be born defective and two in four will also be carriers of the defective gene, a tubal ligation (sterilization) for the woman might be condoned by the Church. Although this point is still debatable among the clergy, there seems to be a trend in this direction. Such a couple should seek counseling through a Catholic social service agency as well as from their physician. If there is a consensus of opinion that the couple should not have children of their own, the woman should then go to the medical ethics committee of a Catholic hospital and request approval for a tubal ligation. Since there is no unanimity among Catholics on this point, the woman might wish to present her case at a second hospital should the first not give approval. In any case, since there is a relaxing of authority against the use of contraceptives, a high-risk couple should be able to avoid an unwanted pregnancy. However, should such a pregnancy occur, and should amniocentesis reveal that the fetus is indeed defective, the couple would have to make the decision whether or not to terminate the pregnancy. In such a case, the Church would probably not condone abortion. The mother would either have to give birth to a defective child or risk excommunication from the Church. In view of the human suffering and tragedy involved for the parents and the child himself, this is truly unfortunate.

One of the world's fastest-growing denominations, the Church of Jesus Christ of Latter-day Saints, known also as the Mormon Church, is opposed in principle to limiting the size of a family merely for the convenience of the parents. According to Mormon principles, one of the main purposes of marriage is to raise a family. However, the Mormons differ from the Catholics in that, in the Mormon faith, each individual interprets the principles of the religion for himself. He is also encouraged to follow the advice of his physician. In the light of this, it would not be morally wrong for a Mormon to use contraceptives to protect the mother's health or to prevent the birth of an abnormal child by having an abortion performed.

For Jewish couples a discussion of birth control and abortion is very important because of the prevalence of Tay-Sachs Disease among Jews. Some people of the Jewish faith oppose abortion and the use of contraceptives, but these are a small minority. The Talmud contains the principles by which the Jew lives; there is no infallible person, such as the Pope, to interpret the Talmud and its legal tradition for the benefit of all Jews; each individual rabbi has his own interpretation and there is a great deal of variation.

The Reform Jews, who are the most liberal, would not oppose birth control or abortion to prevent the birth of a defective child. Although the subject of abortion is controversial among Orthodox Jews, it appears that most of them would also favor terminating a pregnancy to prevent the birth of an abnormal child. Two of the largest Orthodox synagogues in Baltimore have sponsored Tay-Sachs Disease screening programs. Dr. Michael Kaback, who developed the test for determining Tay-Sachs Disease carriers and Tay-Sachs Disease in utero by amniocentesis, found in a survey in Baltimore in 1969 that nearly all the Jewish women surveyed would favor abortion if they knew that they were carrying a fetus with Tay-Sachs Disease. Most of the women stated that they considered abortion under these circumstances to be a personal and medical problem, rather than a religious one, and that in such a case they would consult a doctor rather than their rabbi.

The Hasidic Jews, however, abide very strictly by the rule of the Talmud, which, taken literally, opposes abortion. Although there is variation even among Hasidic Jews, it is likely that a rabbi, if consulted, would object to an abortion under any circumstance. But the Talmud does say that a devoted Jew who reads and studies the Talmud may interpret it for himself, and it would seem that a Jewish woman can choose with a clear conscience to end her pregnancy rather than bear a child who would suffer progressive degeneration, mental retardation, blindness and death within a few years.

Since the legalization of abortion by the Supreme Court, there have been determined efforts to overturn this decision. If these efforts are successful, the result would be a giant step backward in the field of prevention of mental retardation. Those people who advocate an end to legalized abortion often talk about the right to life. In the opinion of the authors, once a child is born he has the right to life, no matter what abnormalities he may have. In addition, he should have a right to a great deal more. He should have a right to a balanced diet and freedom from poverty and prejudice. He should have the right to have his deformities and abnormalities corrected through good medical care. He should have the right not to be locked up against his will in an institution. He should have the right to develop his fullest potential and the right to dignity and self-respect. However, for parents to knowingly bring severely defective children into the world seems irresponsible. The use of abortion to prevent the birth of a child with severe mental retardation is a lifesaving measure rather than a destructive one. If it were not for the option of abortion, a couple producing a child with a severe defect would probably never have another child. In years past, this was often the case. Such couples were deprived of the pleasure of raising healthy, normal children because of the fear that they would produce another defective child. Thanks to the development of amniocentesis and legalized abortion, many children are actually living today who would never have been conceived in former years. High-risk couples are increasingly using these methods of guaranteeing that their child will not suffer from a hereditary form of mental retardation.

Abortion should never be forced upon anyone. If a fetus is found to be abnormal, the decision must be left to the couple involved. And should the couple decide against abortion, their decision must be respected, and they should be assured that their child will receive the best of medical care.

An exciting new avenue in the field of prevention of mental retardation has been opened by the new developments of amniocentesis for detecting severe defects in utero, cytogenetics for examining the chromosomes of the fetal cells, mass screening programs for detecting treatable disorders and thereby preventing mental retardation, and immunizations against common illnesses and for Rh incompatibility. As research continues, more causes will be identified and more treatments developed. The desperate need now is for the medical profession and the public to take advantage of these advancements so that thousands of people can avoid the tragedy and heartbreak of giving birth to a retarded child.

IV
Heredity and Mental Retardation

Although it is known that more than a hundred and sixty different disorders are associated with or cause mental retardation, specific causes are, for the most part, unknown. This fact has been frustrating to both the medical profession and the parents of retarded children. When a child is found to be mentally retarded, the first thing parents want to know is what caused the defect. But it has been estimated that only one quarter of the cases of mental retardation can be traced to known causes. So in most cases the parents must be satisfied with the explanation that this is an accident of nature.

Although much remains to be learned, scientists do know that the causes of mental retardation fall into four different categories: hereditary (genetic), prenatal (before birth), neonatal (from birth to six weeks of age), and post-natal (after six weeks of age). It used to be assumed that most forms of mental retardation were the fault of one of the parents. At the present time, however, scientists believe that only about 20 percent of mental retardation results from hereditary causes.

In order to understand the hereditary causes of mental retardation, it is important to understand the basic construction of the body cells, chromosomes and genes, how they function, and what occurs when an ovum (egg) is fertilized by a sperm cell, and a new individual begins to form.

The human body is made up of cells, each containing a nucleus of chromatin material which consists of 46 tiny rodlike structures called chromosomes. Each chromosome, in turn, contains sixty thousand to eighty thousand genes. These minute genes are the forecasters of the formation of the human body: they contain the sets of instructions which determine whether a person will be tall or short, whether he will have dark or light hair, and in the case of inherited intelligence, whether he will be gifted, average or retarded.

The science of genetics has to do with the study of these genes and their effect on living organisms. Although scientists have been studying human cells through microscopes for years, it has only been since 1956 that they have actually been able to study the chromosomes. In that year, Dr. Joe Hin Tjio and his colleague, Dr. A. Levan, at the National Institutes of Health in Bethesda, Maryland, discovered a simple technique for separating each chromosome from the others. They definitely established that the correct number of chromosomes for the normal human cell is 46. (The number varies with different species of the animal kingdom. For example, gorillas, chimpanzees and orangutans have 48 chromosomes in each cell.) Dr. Tjio received the Kennedy International Mental Retardation award for this important discovery.

Once scientists were able to identify each chromosome individually, more discoveries were made. In 1957 Dr. R. Turpen and Dr. Jerome Lejeune reported that individuals with Down's syndrome had 47 chromosomes in each cell. It was not long before other abnormalities of chromosome material were reported in relation to other disorders. It was especially interesting that most conditions associated with chromosomal abnormalities were also conditions accompanied by mental retardation.

Forty-four of the chromosomes are called autosomes. These 44 autosomes with their thousands of genes determine such characteristics as complexion, color of eyes and hair, and stature. Two of the chromosomes in each cell are related to the sex of the individual, and are therefore called sex chromosomes. These chromosomes are of two types: one related to femaleness and the other to maleness; they are labeled X and Y respectively because their shapes resemble these letters. Two X chromosomes are present in each cell of every female, and an X and Y chromosome are present in each cell of every male. In normal individuals, the chromosomes occur in pairs. So in normal individuals, there are twenty-two pairs of autosomes and one pair of sex chromosomes.

It is now apparent that many changes in chromosomes can occur, either by accident or by inheritance. For example, a part of a chromosome can simply be missing. This is called a *deletion*. Sometimes part of one chromosome becomes attached to another to form a *translocation*. At other times, a part of a chromosome is turned upside down. This is called an *inversion*. And occasionally half of a pair of chromosomes is missing, resulting in only one chromosome instead of a pair. Sometimes a *trisomy* is formed, in which there are three chromosomes of the same type, rather than a pair in a cell.

When a chromosomal defect, such as a deletion, is severe, the cell usually dies. If, however, the defect is not severe enough to kill the cell, that cell with its chromosomal defect will reproduce itself, resulting in a recessive genetic defect. (Recessive and dominant genes will be discussed in detail later in this chapter.)

These discoveries about chromosomes have provided scientists with clues to the causes of some hereditary defects, but many more discoveries remain to be made. The exact location of various genes on the different chromosomes is an exciting area of research; this achievement will undoubtedly happen in our lifetime. New techniques for the identification of the exact parts of each chromosome have already been described. For many years, geneticists have been mapping the gene locations in the chromosomes of the fruit fly. The chromosomes in this organism are relatively large, and the gene sites are more easily identified. It was through the studies of fruit flies that scientists discovered the harmful effects of radiation on the chromosomes. When the fruit fly chromosomes were irradiated, it was found that the radiation caused breakage and distortion of the chromosomes. This evidence was strengthened after the atomic bombs were dropped on Hiroshima and Nagasaki during World War II. Pregnant women who were exposed to the radiation of the bomb blasts produced babies with a high incidence of microcephaly, a condition associated with severe mental retardation. As a result, doctors are careful not to X-ray the abdomens of women during the first three months of pregnancy. Added research in this area could have significant influence on genetic counseling in the future.

The body cells are duplicating themselves all of the

time. As the hair grows, the hair cells are reproducing themselves; when we cut ourselves, new blood cells soon replace any blood that is lost and new skin cells cover the area of the wound. This type of cell duplication, in which any given type of cell has the ability to reproduce itself is called *mitosis*. In most minor injuries to various body tissues and organs, the cells are able to repair themselves in this way. When the injury is more severe, as in the case with injuries to the brain or spinal cord, or as in the case with a stroke, the affected cells may not be able to completely repair themselves, and the patient may have some residual defect. But in most cases, our cells very quietly and efficiently repair any damages through mitosis.

During the process of human reproduction, a different type of cell reproduction begins. This process of cell division which starts in the reproductive systems of the male and female before conception is called *meiosis*. If the sperm and the ovum each had 46 chromosomes, as do the

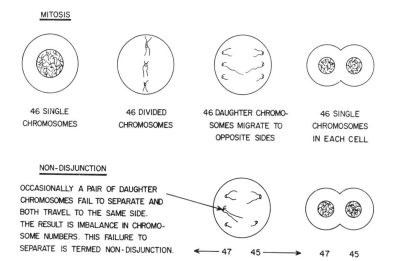

MITOSIS

46 SINGLE CHROMOSOMES

46 DIVIDED CHROMOSOMES

46 DAUGHTER CHROMO- SOMES MIGRATE TO OPPOSITE SIDES

46 SINGLE CHROMOSOMES IN EACH CELL

NON-DISJUNCTION

OCCASIONALLY A PAIR OF DAUGHTER CHROMOSOMES FAIL TO SEPARATE AND BOTH TRAVEL TO THE SAME SIDE. THE RESULT IS IMBALANCE IN CHROMOSOME NUMBERS. THIS FAILURE TO SEPARATE IS TERMED NON-DISJUNCTION.

← 47   45 →   47   45

FERTILIZATION AND ZYGOTE FORMATION

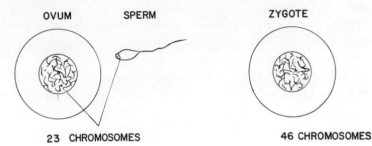

other body cells, their union would produce a cell with 92 chromosomes. However, by an as yet unknown process, the reproductive system of the woman reduces the number of chromosomes while at the same time producing two new ova (eggs). In other words, as two ova are formed, each pair of chromosomes is split, with half going to each of the two ova. Thus for each ovum, there are only 23 chromosomes, one of which is an X or sex chromosome. The male reproductive system also accomplishes this same reduction of chromosomes in its sperm cells. Thus, each of the newly formed sperm cells has 23 chromosomes, but one has the X chromosome and the other has the Y. So at the time of conception, the sperm cell determines whether the new individual will be a male or a female. If the sperm cell which fertilizes the ovum has an X sex chromosome, it will combine with the X of the ovum to produce a girl. If, on the other hand, the sperm cell has the Y sex chromosome, it will combine with the X of the ovum to form an XY, a boy.

Just as accidents can occur in mitosis and produce cells with deletions, inversions and trisomies, resulting in mental retardation, accidents can occur in meiosis cell division. For example, female individuals having only one unpaired X chromosome have been described. These persons are short in stature and outwardly female, but they do not ovulate and thus are sterile. About 20 percent of these women are mentally retarded. Medically, such individuals are said to have Turner's syndrome or, in the new terminology, XO, referring to the fact that they have only one sex chromosome, which is an X. The treatment of such a

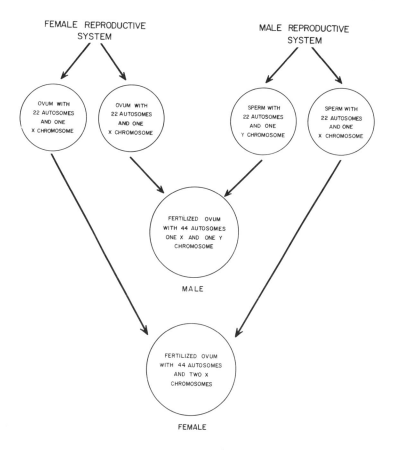

patient would consist of providing extra estrogen, the female hormone produced by the normal ovary. The estrogen improves the physical condition of the patient, but unfortunately, it does not change the mental retardation. Sometimes a male person inherits an extra X chromosome. Such an individual then would have an XXY combination, and is said to have Klinefelter's syndrome. This male person would exhibit breast development and small testes. Sterility is the rule; as yet, no treatment has been established for this defect. About 15 to 20 percent of the patients are also mentally retarded.

As has been explained, during mitosis the sets of instructions (the genes) can duplicate and distribute themselves so that each body cell has the same set of instructions. In other words, when liver cells reproduce, they form other liver cells; blood cells produce other blood cells; and so on. On the other hand, during meiosis, or the cell division which occurs when a new individual is produced, the sperm with its 23 chromosomes containing sixty thousand to eighty thousand genes apiece unites with the egg with its 23 chromosomes and similar number of genes, and at conception the new individual inherits factors from both parents. The new individual will be composed of cells containing sets of instructions derived equally from both contributing parents, but also representing unique combinations of various genes.

How do genetic defects occur? In mitosis, or the duplication of specific types of cells, the genes reproduce themselves generation after generation; therefore the new cells carry the same instructions as were present in their progenitors. Thus, in the genes producing the color component of the tissues (skin, eyes, hair, etc.) the cells are faithful to a certain pattern, such as red hair, fair skin and blue eyes. But occasionally, errors do occur in the reproduction of the genes. These errors may result either in the failure of the production of some enzyme, or in the formation of an enzyme or protein somewhat different from the usual or original one. (An enzyme is a protein substance which has the ability to initiate or speed up many chemical processes in living tissues.) Thus, if at the time of fertilization an error occurred in which the genes governing the color component in skin, hair and eyes were missing, the enzyme to initiate production of this color component would also be missing and the cells would reproduce themselves without color, for the error is as heritable as were the original instructions. This type of error is called a *mutation*. Occasionally we see just such mutations in the human and animal world in the form of albinos, who have very light skin, very blond hair, and eyes which appear pink because of the color of the blood (actually, the eyes are colorless, also). When mutation produces an enzyme similar to the original gene's product, the effect may not be noticeable. Occasionally the new product is better than the old. But sometimes the result of a mutation is a protein so incompatible with the whole system that the organism is unable to live and the fetus is spontaneously aborted; these are called lethal mutations. In between the extremes, there are mutations that seriously disturb normal development of the individual and are thus deleterious, but they do not result in death. In the field of mental retardation, such mutations would account for such disorders as spina bifida and anencephaly. Spina bifida is a condition in which there are defects in the brain and spinal cord, and anencephaly is a disorder in which the major part of the brain is absent.

Occasionally mutation instructions are passed on to another human generation, producing a hereditary defect. Patients suffering serious defects usually do not have children, but there are some serious disorders which are hereditary. PKU (discussed in a later chapter) is an example of a nonlethal but serious hereditary defect caused by a prior mutation. This disorder occurs when a recessive gene causes the absence of certain enzymes which are necessary for the body's proper assimilation of a component of protein. Due to the absence of the enzyme, the protein component phenylalanine builds up in the body and eventually causes brain damage. Fortunately, prompt diagnosis and dietary treatment can prevent the brain damage from occurring, but there is no treatment for the defective gene.

At the time of fertilization, when the sperm cell with its 23 chromosomes unites with the ovum, which also has 23 chromosomes, each chromosome seeks out its proper partner so that the chromosomes are again in pairs, as they are in all other body cells. The two sex chromosomes become a pair, and the other chromosomes, the autosomes, migrate to the appropriate partner to form the normal total of 23 pairs. When this pairing of chromosomes, each with its thousands of genes, takes place, the genes must also work in pairs. Some genes, however, are dominant over others. For example, if two parents have brown eyes and dark hair, the genes governing coloring which are present in the newly fertilized ovum will, for the most part, predestine the new individual to have brown eyes and dark hair. If, however, one of the parents has fair skin, blue eyes and blond hair, and the other has brown eyes and dark skin and dark hair, their offspring will almost invariably have brown eyes and dark skin and dark hair; scientists have discovered that genes carrying instructions for darker coloring are nearly always dominant over genes carrying instructions for lighter coloring. In the example cited, some genetic effect of the light-complexioned parent would exhibit itself, with the offspring having a slightly lighter complexion and hair than the darker parent, unless that parent was of a pure strain and had never had any fair-skinned, blond forebears.

Occasionally there are exceptions to this rule. The genes may arrange themselves in such a fashion that the recessive genes from one parent will combine with the genes of the other parent to produce an offspring who differs from the predictable. For example, the dark-complexioned partner may have had a blond, fair-skinned grandparent. In his genetic makeup, he carries genes for blond hair and fair skin, but these genes are recessive. Most of his genes governing hair and skin color carry the code for dark skin and hair. But in the process of chromosome pairing, the recessive genes of the dark-complexioned partner can by chance be paired with the genes of the light-complexioned partner, producing a blond, fair-skinned offspring, who is an exception to the genetic rule. We have all heard jokes about the red-headed milkman who is under suspicion when a customer, a brunette housewife, gives birth to a red-headed child. But it is quite possible for this to occur without any hanky-panky between the housewife and the milkman.

Dominance and recessiveness were first studied by an Austrian monk, Gregor Mendel, of the Abbey of Brünn, who published a paper in 1866 on his findings. During the seven years between 1856 and 1863, he experimented with pea plants in a portion of the monastery garden. He found that the offspring of a tall, pure strain of pea plant and a short, pure strain of pea plant was always a tall plant. In the pea plant, each cell has only two genes for height; the tall pure strain plant had two genes for tallness, or TT, and the short, pure strain plant had two genes for shortness, or tt. Therefore, the genes for tallness were dominant. But he found that if two of these hybrid (mixed) offspring were mated, one in four of their offspring, on the average, was short. He therefore postulated that the tall strain with its two hereditary factors (genes) for tallness, TT, and the short strain, with its two hereditary factors for shortness, tt, produced offspring with one hereditary factor from each parent, thus having the genetic constitution of Tt, and that such a pea with one hereditary factor for tallness (T) and one for shortness (t) was as tall as one with the genetic constitution TT. He also postulated that when a plant grows reproductive cells, only one member of the pair of height genes passes into any one reproductive cell, and that it is pure chance which it is. This is plant meiosis. Thus, a tall pea plant with a genetic constitution of Tt is equally likely to form reproductive cells with T for tallness, or gene t for shortness. The possible combinations of genes in the offspring can be TT, tT, Tt, or tt. In the tt plants, the two recessive genes have combined, and the plant is short. In other words, one out of four offspring from the two tall plants is short because of recessive genes.

By transposing this much simplified explanation to the human species, it is possible to see how dominant and recessive genes can interact to form many combinations of hereditary factors. In the field of mental retardation, two people who have identical defective recessive genes are at high risk of producing an offspring with a hereditary genetic defect. Some forty to fifty serious disorders which cause mental retardation are passed on in this manner. These diseases are often lethal, with the patients living only a few months or years. However, in cases where the patient survives the physical stresses of the disorder, severe mental retardation nearly always manifests itself. Diseases of this type are said to be due to *metabolic disorders*.

Metabolism refers to the manner in which the body produces energy from food to maintain the life cycle of the body cells. For example, the life span of the average

liver cell is two months; through metabolism the body provides the energy for the process of mitosis, which creates
the liver cell. It then supplies the fuel so that the cell can
function and carry on its work of purifying the blood for
the two months of its life. When the cell dies, through the
metabolic process, the dead cell is recycled and changed
to the various proteins and chemicals of which it is composed, and these components are then absorbed and reused
by the body. The life span of each type of cell is different.
For example, the life span of red blood cells is about two
hundred days, and that of white blood cells is only three
days. Thus the body is constantly producing, maintaining
and recycling cells in this very complicated and delicately
balanced process.

Any disease which interferes with the process of
metabolism is called a metabolic disease. One such disease
is galactosemia, in which the sugar called galactose is not
properly used by the body because of a missing enzyme.
Instead of being changed to glucose, which the body needs,
the galactose accumulates in the blood and body tissues in
large amounts, and is eventually excreted in the urine. It
causes such physical symptoms as nausea, vomiting and
weight loss, and it also usually causes mental retardation.
Another metabolic disorder which is caused by a recessive
genetic defect is maple syrup urine disease, in which a
protein is not properly assimilated by the body. In this disorder, as in galactosemia, a substance which the normal
system needs cannot be broken down for proper use, and,
instead, builds up in the tissues and bloodstream, eventually causing brain damage. In maple syrup urine disease,
it is a protein which cannot be properly metabolized. As
the name suggests, one of the symptoms of the disorder is
the fact that the patient's urine smells like maple syrup. The
metabolic diseases all have several things in common. The

patients are unable to use some substance—a fat, a protein or a sugar—which is needed and utilized by the normal person, and they nearly always become severely mentally retarded.

It is in this field that researchers are making a great deal of progress. Although some of these disorders are rare, they are all diagnosable. In some cases the carriers of the genetic defect can be diagnosed. Thus it should be possible with proper diagnosis and genetic counseling to completely eliminate the disease. Any time such a disorder is diagnosed, the close relatives of the patient should be studied to determine which ones are the carriers of the defect. The usual method of detection is a blood or urine test. The carriers of the defect should be informed so that when they marry, their partners can be tested to make sure they do not carry identical genetic defects. If both partners are found to have the same defect, they should be counseled not to have children of their own. However, if only one of them exhibited the defect the normal gene of the other partner would be dominant in their offspring, and therefore there would be no need for worry. In some diseases where the carriers cannot be determined, amniocentesis (test of amniotic fluid during early pregnancy) can reveal the presence of the disorder in a fetus. In such a case, the fetus could be aborted. In any case, when such a hereditary disorder is diagnosed, it is very important for the family to be referred to a good genetic counseling center. Such services are to be found at all medical schools and at some state health departments.

For many years the medical profession has been aware that certain diseases are inherited because of defects in the sex chromosomes. These are called sex-linked diseases. The best-known example of a sex-linked hereditary disease is hemophilia, the blood disease which plagued the Bourbon dynasty of Europe during the eighteenth and nine-teenth centuries. In recent years, four disorders causing mental retardation have been shown to be sex-linked. They are oculo-cerebral-renal disease, Hunter's Disease, kinky hair disease, and axonal dysplasia. Oculo-cerebral-renal disease is caused by a metabolic defect in which certain protein substances cannot be properly assimilated. The patient develops eye cataracts, poor muscle tone, and men-tal retardation. Hunter's Disease is a sex-linked form of gargoylism in which the stature is dwarfed, and there is a shortness of the neck and trunk and a clouding of the corneas of the eyes. Kinky hair disease is a metabolic dis-order in which the body is unable to properly utilize cop-per. Two of the symptoms are kinky hair and profound mental retardation. In axonal dysplasia, the patient suffers convulsions, severe mental retardation and nerve degenera-tion. Unfortunately, there is no known treatment for these diseases at the present time, and the patients usually die in early childhood. Here again, genetic counseling can help the parents avoid much expense and heartbreak.

In these sex-linked diseases, a definite pattern of inheritance ensues. By studying this pattern, geneticists have established the fact that the female carries a defective gene on one of her two X chromosomes. Since she is per-fectly normal, she probably never realizes that she is a carrier until she marries and bears children; on the average, half of her sons will be victims of the disease, and half of her daughters will also be carriers. It may seem impossible that a person can be perfectly normal and yet carry a defective gene, but this can occur if the defective gene is recessive. Thus, the female is normal because the defective gene on one of her X chromosomes is dominated by the appropriate gene on her other X chromosome. This leaves her free from the disease, but when she bears children the defective gene will be passed on. Some of her daughters will also become carriers and some of her sons will suffer from the disease. This is explained by the fact that her sons will inherit an X chromosome from her and a Y chromosome from their father; therefore approximately half of her sons will inherit the chromosome with the defect. Since males have the XY sex-chromosome pair, if there is a defect on the X chromosome there is no corresponding gene on the Y chromosome to dominate it, so that the male inherits the disease. The disease cannot be passed on by the affected male, since his defective gene, which is always on his X chromosome, will always be dominated in his offspring by the corresponding gene on the chromosome of his partner. The only time such a disease can pass from a father to his children is when the affected male marries a female who is herself a carrier of the same disease. In such a case, among their offspring, on the average, half of the males will inherit the disease, half of the females will also inherit the disease, and the rest of the females will be carriers.

For many years, intelligence was thought to be a fixed, inherent quality of the human organism. Genetic factors were thought to be all-important. In fact, for several decades, sterilization was practiced widely in certain state institutions for the retarded. On the surface, this may appear to have been a good solution, as it is known that mentally retarded parents are more likely to produce mentally retarded children. However, with advancements in the field of diagnosis and treatment, it has been found that some people of normal intelligence were placed in institutions for the retarded, and consequently sterilized. Most of them had been thought to be retarded because they suffered from other defects, such as deafness, which made them appear retarded. When it was found that they had normal intelligence, they were released from the institutions, but, of course, they were sterile. Physicians and geneticists now feel that selective sterilization after thorough diagnosis and study is a wiser procedure than indiscriminate sterilization. Of special importance in combating hereditary diseases is good genetic counseling.

> One minute chromosome—
> So small and intricate—
> It can't even be seen
> By the naked eye; yet so
> Omnipotent, it may determine
> One's destiny . . .
>
> *Christine Koch*

V
Prenatal Causes of Mental Retardation

The period of time between the fertilization of the ovum and the delivery of the baby is known as the prenatal period. Immediately after fertilization, the ovum implants itself in the thick lining of the uterus where it begins a period of rapid growth during which it develops human form, and at the end of nine months emerges as a living individual.

During the first few weeks, the embryo is nourished by the thick lining cells of the uterus. At the site of implantation, a mass of blood vessels and tissue cells form to supply the growing demands of the embryo. This sponge-like mass develops into the placenta, which acts as a sort of middleman between the mother and the new individual forming within her. It not only provides nourishment and oxygen for the embryo, but it protects it by screening out certain infectious agents, such as viruses and bacteria, which might otherwise be transferred to it from the mother.

As the placenta grows, the embryo moves away from the uterine wall, leaving only the placenta at the site of implantation. At the same time, the umbilical cord forms between the embryo and the placenta through which the life-giving nourishment and oxygen are supplied to the developing baby. And as the embryo grows and moves away from the uterine wall, it becomes surrounded by a protective bag of water, the amniotic fluid. Thus the body of the mother supplies the needs for the protection and growth of a healthy new individual.

This initial phase is a critical period for the developing embryo. As early as the eighteenth day of pregnancy, the cells of the embryo are beginning to arrange themselves in layers which will form the structures of the body. During this stage of development, the embryo is very vulnerable to adverse conditions. It can be severely damaged by infections, the use of certain drugs by the mother, malnutrition or illness of the mother, iron deficiency of the mother, radiation, injury or lack of oxygen. Toxemia of pregnancy and blood incompatibility can also be devastating to the embryo. Maternal emotional instability may also interfere with the development of the embryo, although evidence in support of this is scanty. In essence, any factor causing maternal ill health may have an adverse effect on the unborn child.

Although the placenta provides protection for the fetus, it is not able to filter out all infectious agents. Since the organisms which cause bacterial infections are quite large, they are usually screened out by the placenta, but occasionally they do reach the unborn child. Virus infections are caused by smaller organisms, however, and they are more easily transmitted to the fetus. Some diseases may be so damaging to the unborn infant as to cause its death, resulting in a spontaneous abortion. Others, less severe, may not kill the fetus, but may result in the child's being born with a defect. Such an abnormality which is present at birth is called a congenital defect.

Before the advent of antibiotics, syphilis was a common infection causing congenital defects. This disease caused prematurity, keratitis (an infection of the outer covering of the eyeball), rhagades (a deformity of the mouth), snuffles (chronic nasal discharge), and bony changes caused by the fact that the infection had invaded the bone ends. The infection also attacked the nervous system, causing mental defect. Fortunately, with compulsory premarital and prenatal tests for syphilis, as well as adequate penicillin therapy, this form of brain damage is rare today.

Toxoplasmosis is a disease about which not much is known. It is usually undiagnosed in the general population, yet nearly one third of the population carries antibodies to this protozoan organism, indicating that they have been exposed to it at some time. When a mother contracts this disease early in pregnancy, congenital defects involving the central nervous system may occur in her developing baby. The manner of infection is not definitely known, but raw meat is known to be a carrier. It is thought that there are other important avenues of spreading toxoplasmosis, since it occurs throughout the United States. An infant infected by toxoplasmosis may exhibit serious defects of the choroid membrane (part of the vascular system of the eye) and the central nervous system. Skull X-rays may reveal calcium deposits in the brain. Mental defect and convulsions usually occur. Unfortunately, there is as yet no therapy of proven value. This condition accounts for less than one percent of the mentally retarded. The diagnosis can be confirmed by antibody studies on the mother and a positive skin test on the affected child.

Whereas the danger posed to pregnant women by bacterial infections has been greatly reduced by the advent of antibiotics, this, unfortunately, is not true of viral infections. As mentioned before, viruses are smaller than bacteria, and they seem able to pass through the placenta more easily than bacteria can.

One of the most dangerous viruses during pregnancy is the rubella virus. It was not until 1941 that the relationship between rubella (German or three-day-measles) in pregnant women and congenital defects in their offspring was reported in medical literature. Subsequent studies have revealed that if the mother has rubella during her first month of pregnancy she runs a 50 percent risk of having an affected child. If the infection occurs during the second month of pregnancy, the risk is reduced to 22 percent, and during the third month the risk declines to 6 percent. If the infection occurs later in the pregnancy, the fetus may become infected without suffering an abnormality; however, the rubella virus may be found in its system for many months after birth. Such an infant can even spread the disease because the virus lives and multiplies in its kidneys and is excreted in the urine.

The types of congenital abnormalities caused by this virus are both physical and mental. They include low birth weight, eye defects, such as cataracts and glaucoma, deafness, microcephaly, heart abnormality, skin rash, jaundice and mental retardation.

In 1958 Dr. Saul Krugman and Dr. Robert Ward found that gamma globulin prevented the symptoms of rubella, and gamma globulin shots were administered to most pregnant women who knew they had been exposed to the disease. This treatment did not prove to be completely successful, however. Although research with gamma globulin and rubella continues, it appears now that although gamma globulin does prevent the rubella symptoms in the mother, she does become infected by the virus and the treatment does not always prevent the infection from being transmitted to the embryo and producing the abnormalities.

The development of the rubella vaccine should have provided excellent control of this disease but it has not, because many people have not taken advantage of this method of immunization. Doctors are fearful of using the vaccine for any woman who might be pregnant, and still rely to a great extent on the less reliable gamma globulin treatment in cases where pregnant women have been exposed to the disease. The situation would be improved if doctors with adolescent girl patients would stress the importance of the rubella immunization.

A number of other viral diseases have been suspected of causing abnormalities in unborn infants. They are very rare, however, and it has not been definitely proven that they do actually cause defects. It is sufficient to say here that expectant mothers should avoid contact with infections such as regular measles, mumps, chicken pox and hepatitis. They should check with their doctors if any illnesses occur during pregnancy.

Another prenatal cause of mental retardation is hormonal imbalance. This form of defect is not commonly found in the United States at this time, since it is usually related to having an inadequate amount of iodine in the diet. Most Americans who have an inadequate amount of iodine in their drinking water use iodized salt. In some of the underdeveloped parts of the world, such as the Andes region in South America where there is a lack of iodine in the diet and where the people do not have access to iodized salt, occasionally women develop goiters, which are a symptom of thyroid deficiency. These women often give birth to cretins. Cretinism is a disorder caused by an absence of thyroid hormone, which is necessary for proper physical and mental growth. Victims of this disorder are small in stature, have rough, dry skin and dry, sparse hair, and are mentally retarded. Cretinism can be successfully treated by the administration of thyroid extract to the infant if the defect is discovered before mental retardation has become pronounced.

Chronic maternal illnesses always pose added risks to the unborn child. Women who suffer from such disorders as high blood pressure, kidney disease and diabetes should be under good medical care during their pregnancy. Some of these illnesses can cause physical disorders, such as heart disease, among the infants, and others can cause mental retardation. For example, in maternal PKU, if the mother does not observe her special dietary restrictions, the elevated level of phenylalanine in her system can cause damage to the developing brain of her baby.

Mental retardation has also been seen in children of mothers who develop untreated pernicious anemia. This is a disease in which vitamin B_{12} is not absorbed properly. Scientists therefore believe that a lack of vitamin B_{12} is damaging to the central nervous system of the unborn child. Studies with animals have shown that there is an increased risk of abnormalities of various types due to maternal vitamin deficiencies. It seems logical to assume that maternal malnutrition would cause mental retardation in the offspring, but there is as yet no actual proof that it does.

The use of various kinds of drugs during pregnancy

can also cause brain damage, as well as other abnormalities in the unborn child. The most recent example is that of the drug thalidomide; although the infants born to women who used this drug during pregnancy were not mentally retarded, they were born with severe malformations of the arms and legs. Some antimetabolic drugs, such as those used in the treatment of cancer, cause many abnormalities, including mental retardation; they also cause miscarriage. Overuse of insulin by the mother during pregnancy can also cause brain damage in the infant. Excessive cigarette smoking by the mother has already been mentioned as a cause of the abnormal smallness of newborn infants. Doctors have found, as a general rule, that the lower the birth weight, the greater is the possibility of mental retardation.

As has been mentioned earlier, radiation of the fetus within three months of conception is harmful. In the 1930's some pregnant women were treated by X-ray therapy for cancer of the uterus; they produced children who were microcephalic (having small heads and small brains) and had other defects. Needless to say, this treatment is no longer used during pregnancy.

Anoxia can also cause mental retardation in the unborn infant. Anoxia refers to a lack of oxygen. This can occur if the mother suffers a near drowning or an accidental suffocation. It can also be caused by carbon monoxide poisoning. The lack of oxygen for the unborn child in such circumstances can produce brain damage or a convulsive disorder. It is of historical interest that Julius Caesar, who was a man of many unusual abilities, suffered from a convulsive disorder. History tells us that he was born by a Caesarean operation as his mother lay dying; therefore he may have suffered anoxia at birth, and this would explain the cause of the convulsions.

Injury to the abdomen of the mother could cause

premature separation of the placenta from the uterine wall. In such a case, the infant would suffer anoxia. This could also cause a premature delivery. Although there is no clear evidence to prove the supposition, it seems logical that severe injury to the abdomen of the mother could damage the fetus. Damage can also be caused to the fetus when foreign objects are introduced into the uterus. In the past, women sometimes did this to try to induce an abortion. The incidence of such cases is decreasing with the advent of more effective birth control methods and liberalized abortion laws.

Emotional stress may also be a factor in the birth of infants who suffer abnormalities. Although it is difficult to gather scientific data on this problem, it is reasonable to assume that any severe stress, whether mental or physical, can affect the unborn infant, and that the healthier the pregnancy in all aspects, the better the chance there is for the newborn baby to be normal.

One of the major causes of mental retardation is prematurity. This condition alone accounts for 24.5 percent of all deaths among newborn infants, and it is associated with 15 to 20 percent of all cases of mental retardation. Infants are classified by weight to determine whether or not they are premature. Babies weighing less than 2500 grams (5 pounds and 8 ounces) at birth are considered to be premature. In some South American countries, where there is a significant amount of maternal malnutrition, this figure is thought to range between 2200 to 2300 grams. Chances are excellent that infants weighing more than 2000 grams will survive and be normal, but the probability of survival drops to 10 percent when the infant weighs less than 1000 grams (a little over a pound). Doctors do not know why there is a relationship between the weight of the infant and his ability to survive and be normal, but it is thought that it is because certain of the body tissues of the premature infant are immature and unable to perform their necessary tasks. It follows, then, that the greater the degree of prematurity, the greater the chance of abnormality. The premature infant is a delicate, unfinished creature. Two disorders which are especially related to prematurity are neonatal atelectasis and hyaline membrane disease. In neonatal atelectasis, the lungs of the newborn infant fail to expand with air; this, of course, can result in anoxia and brain damage. Hyaline membrane disease is also related to the inability of the respiratory system of the premature infant to function normally. Liver immaturity is also a serious problem. If the liver is unable to handle its many tasks, the infant may become jaundiced. Such an infant develops a yellow coloring to his skin which is caused by a bile pigment, bilirubin, which is not properly metabolized when the liver is immature. This condition interferes with the use of oxygen by the body cells; therefore, when it becomes severe the child may suffer damage such as deafness, athetosis (abnormal, involuntary hand and wrist movements) and mental retardation.

Prematurity is often caused by the occurrence of twins. In such a case, the second twin born is at a greater risk, since it must endure longer labor. In addition, the placenta may separate from the infant when the first twin is born, and since the placenta is the unborn infant's only source of oxygen, premature separation from the placenta can cause mental retardation and even death.

Often premature births occur because the mother is suffering from some illness, such as Rh incompatibility or toxemia of pregnancy.

Rh incompatibility refers to a blood condition which can have serious consequences for the baby. The Rh factor is a substance which is present on the surface of the red blood cells of some individuals but is absent in others. A person having the Rh factor on his red blood cells is said to be Rh positive, while one having no Rh factor is Rh negative. Eighty-five percent of the population is Rh positive and the other 15 percent is Rh negative. The offspring of two Rh positive parents will, of course, be Rh positive, and the offspring of two Rh negative parents will be Rh negative. Both the Rh positive and the Rh negative individuals are perfectly healthy and normal. The offspring of an Rh positive mother and an Rh negative father will be Rh positive because the Rh factor is dominant. But if the father is Rh positive and the mother is Rh negative, the fetus will be Rh positive—which means that the blood of the mother and the fetus will be incompatible, the mother being Rh negative and the fetus, Rh positive. Although the mother and the fetus have separate circulatory systems and their blood does not mix, a few blood cells from the fetus get through the placenta and enter the circulatory system of the mother, and in like manner a few of the mother's blood cells enter the circulatory system of the fetus.

In the case of the Rh negative mother and the Rh positive fetus, when the few blood cells of the fetus escape into the circulatory system of the mother, her body starts to produce antibodies to the Rh factor which is foreign to her system. These antibodies have the ability to destroy the offending Rh positive red blood cells, causing them to break down into protein, iron and hemoglobin. For the duration of the pregnancy, the mother's body continues to produce these antibodies, which readily pass through the placenta and attack the red blood cells in the system of the fetus. As a result of the breakdown of large numbers of red blood cells within the fetus, bilirubin is produced within its system. The bilirubin has such a toxic effect, by interfering with the oxygen supply of the fetus, that the infant can suffer permanent brain damage. In severe cases the fetus becomes so anemic from the loss of red blood cells and weak from the toxic bilirubin in its system that it dies before birth. In some cases, these babies are born prematurely, alive, but in a weakened condition.

Beginning in 1951, exchange transfusions were performed on babies born with the Rh problem in which all of their blood was completely replaced by Rh negative blood. If this was done immediately after birth, usually the infant could be saved from mental retardation, but without the exchange transfusion the antibodies in the newborn infant continued to destroy the red blood cells, with mental retardation almost a certainty.

There has been a dramatic new development in cases of Rh blood incompatibility. An immunization to the antibodies was recently developed in Australia. Thus, an Rh negative woman whose husband is Rh positive can be immunized before her body reacts to the Rh factor and no antibodies will be formed. This procedure has proven perfectly safe, causing no adverse reaction whatever in the mother, and it completely circumvents the severe complications of Rh blood incompatibility. This immunization should be given after the birth of the first child. The State of California now has a law making it mandatory that prenatal tests include an evaluation of the Rh factor in all pregnant women. Another cause of premature births is toxemia, a disease of pregnancy which needs more study. The severe consequences of unrecognized and untreated toxemia to the mother and the unborn child have already been discussed. This disorder accounts for one third of all maternal deaths. Toxemia can result in a premature delivery, with the resulting greater risk to the baby; it has also been suggested that even when carried to full term, babies born of mothers with untreated toxemia are less likely to be normal than other babies. This is certainly true in severe cases where the mother has suffered convulsions and coma. This condition can be treated by the restriction of salt in the mother's diet, rest and sedation. In severe cases, where the mother does not respond to treatment, obstetricians often try to induce labor early, or they deliver the child early by Caesarean operation.

Intrauterine growth retardation (Warkany's Syndrome) is another condition that is poorly understood. This disease is characterized by an abnormally small placenta and the low birth weight of the infant, in spite of the fact that the pregnancy has lasted the normal nine-month period. These infants have small heads, prominent noses and underdeveloped lower jaws; they are generally small in stature and mentally retarded. This condition occurs in approximately one out of every 1,000 pregnancies.

Recent animal research has demonstrated that protein deficiency during pregnancy may also cause mental retardation, since it leads to intrauterine stunting and impaired brain development. According to estimates made by the President's Committee on Mental Retardation, 50 percent of the women in large urban areas suffer from protein malnutrition. In addition, many rural populations suffer severe lack of protein. This means that there is risk of malnutrition in 350,000 pregnancies per year in this country.

The President's Committee also points out that since malnutrition is totally preventable, every effort should be made to eliminate this factor as a cause of mental retardation. The estimated cost of protein supplementation is small (ten to twenty dollars per pregnancy). Powdered milk, calcium, iron and vitamins would provide an adequate dietary supplement in most cases. Thus, in an area such as Los Angeles County, where there are approximately 10,500 births annually to women receiving welfare, the cost of such a program would be about $210,000, less than the cost of lifetime institutional care for a single retarded person ($250,000). If severe retardation were prevented in only two cases per year, the taxpayers would save money.

A program such as this could be operated as it is in England, where pregnant women are entitled to obtain milk, calcium, iron and vitamins at their local health department. This program has an added advantage in that a woman registering for the food supplement is given regular examinations to ensure that her pregnancy is normal and healthy. In this way, many women who would not otherwise have any prenatal care receive good medical monitoring of their pregnancies.

The United States has a higher rate of infant mortality associated with prenatal complications than do most of the other developed countries of the world. It is reprehensible that this should be so in such a wealthy nation.

VI
Birth Injuries

At the end of the prenatal period the fetus is very low in the uterus. Usually, a few days before the onset of labor the child's head actually drops down into the pelvis. In medical terms, the head becomes "engaged."

With the onset of labor, the muscles of the uterus begin to contract and push the child out of the cervical canal. At the same time, the tissue surrounding the amniotic fluid ruptures and the fluid gradually escapes, providing lubrication which helps the child move down the cervical canal. With the contractions of labor, the muscles of the cervix (outlet of the uterus) dilate until the infant, followed by the umbilical cord, is pushed through the cervix and out of the vagina. The placenta (afterbirth) usually delivers within five or ten minutes after the birth of the baby.

The process of labor can last for only a few minutes, or it can take many hours or even several days. The speed at which labor proceeds can be important to the health of both the mother and the baby. The labor for a first child is usually longer and harder than it is for subsequent births; the average length of a first labor is eighteen hours. Prolonged labor may indicate a number of problems, such as uterine inertia, pelvic abnormality, the baby's having an excessively large head or large body or being abnormally positioned. An excessively long labor can result in maternal exhaustion or in anoxia of the baby.

On the other hand, a very rapid labor and delivery can also be harmful. During the process of birth, the baby's head slowly molds to the shape of the confining bones of the pelvis. During a precipitous delivery the head molds and then reexpands very rapidly. Because of this swift constriction and expansion, the capillary blood vessels in the baby's head can rupture, causing hemorrhage into the brain. This is usually followed by scarring of the brain tissue and brain damage.

Birth injury resulting either in bleeding into the brain or in anoxia was formerly a common cause of mental retardation, but modern obstetrical methods have reduced these threats. Statistics from the Mental Retardation Clinic at Childrens Hospital of Los Angeles show that only 5 percent of the retarded children evaluated have conditions related to birth injury.

In the past, forceps deliveries were thought to be the cause of many birth injuries, but it is now felt that these injuries were probably due to either a very long, hard labor or a very precipitous delivery. Low-forceps deliveries are those in which the baby's head is merely helped out of the birth canal; such use of forceps can actually minimize the chance of birth injury. The use of the instrument when the baby is midway down the birth canal is called a mid-forceps delivery, and that of bringing the baby's head down into the pelvis is a high-forceps delivery. Mid- and high-forceps deliveries are seldom necessary, and should be performed only by a skilled obstetrician.

The position of the baby in the uterus is important in the birth process. Usually the baby is born head first, which presents an easier delivery than any other position. About 3 percent of babies are born in a breech position (buttocks first). Because the umbilical cord can easily become compressed between the mother's pelvis and the baby's head during such a delivery, anoxia and brain damage occur more frequently in a breech delivery. A transverse position is the most serious. In such a case, an arm or shoulder may present first, with the baby's body lodged across the opening of the birth canal. When the baby is in this position, delivery is virtually impossible. Before the advent of modern obstetrics, neither the mother nor the infant survived a transverse delivery. Today, the infant is actually turned by the obstetrician to afford a breech delivery, or a Caesarean operation is performed. This procedure must be done skillfully and promptly to avoid danger of brain damage to the infant.

Another complication during a delivery which poses danger for the mother and infant is the result of prior surgical procedures involving the uterus. In Caesarean operations, the wall of the uterus is cut open so that the infant can be removed. After such an operation, the muscles of the uterus wall are not as strong as they were before surgery because of the scar tissue at the site of the incision. In such a case, there would be danger of the uterus rupturing during any subsequent labor. If this occurred, the mother would go into shock and suffer massive hemorrhage. The infant would then suffer anoxia due to the loss of blood. For this reason, after a woman has given birth by Caesarean or has had surgery involving the uterus, subsequent deliveries are usually made by Caesarean operation.

There can also be complications because of the location of the placenta. The ovum usually implants in the upper part of the uterus, but occasionally it implants over the cervix (opening of the womb). With the onset of labor in such a case, the placenta, which forms at the site of implantation, separates from the wall of the uterus. This condition is called *placenta previa*. In situations where there has been no prenatal care, cases of placenta previa nearly always result in cerebral damage to the infant because of anoxia during delivery. In order to supply oxygen to the infant during delivery and until the baby begins breathing on its own, the placenta must remain attached to the uterine wall during the birth process. In placenta previa, the baby is without oxygen during the delivery. When this condition is present, there is usually a slight bloody discharge during the latter stages of the pregnancy. With good obstetrical care, placenta previa can be diagnosed before the onset of labor, and the baby delivered by Caesarean operation.

In rare cases, the placenta separates prematurely from the uterus. This condition is called *placenta abruptio*. If the resulting hemorrhage is not detected, the mother may go into shock and the infant may die. When this condition occurs the mother's blood pressure drops immediately, so if her labor is being carefully monitored a Caesarean operation can be performed immediately. If there is undue delay the infant may suffer anoxia and brain damage through loss of blood.

Complications can also arise during delivery because

of abnormalities in the umbilical cord. Occasionally the cord may not be the proper length. If it is too short, it may rupture during labor and cause hemorrhaging. If it is too long, it may turn on itself and precede the baby at the birth canal; the cord becomes compressed between the child's head and the pelvic bones during delivery and causes anoxia in the infant. This condition is referred to as a prolapse of the cord, and fortunately it is unusual.

In the past, many women suffered pelvic deformity as a result of rickets. This threat has declined in recent years, but automobile accidents have created a new and increasing cause of pelvic deformity. A woman who has suffered a broken pelvis may have enough deformity to cause a prolonged labor during which the baby may suffer anoxia; in such a case, a Caesarean operation is usually performed before the onset of labor. For expectant mothers with this problem, a detailed medical history and good obstetrical care are important.

The neonatal period refers to the period between birth and six weeks of age. A variety of symptoms may be present during the neonatal period, and it is important to have a pediatrician evaluate the baby's physical status. Some conditions may be of little consequence, but others may indicate serious problems which need immediate attention in order to prevent or minimize permanent damage. A number of these symptoms may be associated with brain injury or abnormality. A baby who does not breathe spontaneously or whose breathing is irregular, and who has poor sucking and cough reflexes, may have a brain abnormality accompanied by mental retardation.

It is important to know that some infants may display abnormal symptoms at birth without suffering permanent damage. For example, such neurological signs as lethargy, spasticity (increased muscle tone) and abnormal hand patterns do not necessarily predict trouble in later life. A recent study indicates that even an abnormal electroencephalogram obtained during the newborn period has little prognostic value. In other words, neurological signs and electroencephalogram results during this period may be considered among other things to help a diagnostician obtain a clear picture. But these findings should only be considered as a part of the overall picture, and not as an all-important indication of damage.

Convulsions are not uncommon during the newborn period and may result from a number of causes. It is thought that intracranial hemorrhage is the most common cause, and in many cases is an indication of brain injury. Convulsions during this period may also be caused by infections of the brain due to organisms such as viruses and bacteria. These infections can actually destroy brain tissue and, of course, cause retardation. Prompt antibiotic treatment usually minimizes the chances of brain damage occurring.

Another condition which can cause convulsions and brain damage during the newborn period is *hypoglycemia* (low blood sugar). Glucose (blood sugar) is the source of fuel for brain energy. When there is a lack of glucose for the brain, convulsions and brain damage can result. There are a variety of possible causes for this condition, including thyroid disease, metabolic diseases, tumors of the pancreas and starvation, but for the most part the actual causes of this disorder are unknown. The symptoms can be treated by the use of a diet high in protein and carbohydrates. The outlook for children suffering from hypoglycemia differs, depending upon the severity of the symptoms. Usually the disease becomes less severe as the child grows older, but repeated convulsions due to hypoglycemia usually cause brain damage.

A condition similar in some respects to convulsions is *tetany*, in which the baby's muscles are flexed and rigid. Unlike a convulsion, which subsides spontaneously, tetany can be relieved only by the administration of calcium. If this condition is prolonged and untreated, it can result in brain damage.

Until recent years, pediatricians saw numerous cases of cerebral palsy and other forms of brain damage during the neonatal period which were caused by poor obstetrics, Rh blood incompatibility, inadequate care of premature infants and other neonatal complications. In large measure, these are no longer seen. Fortunately, modern medical care is significantly reducing the incidence of mental retardation due to injuries and disorders associated with the birth process. Obstetricians are no longer fearful of performing Caesarean operations now that antibiotics have reduced the risk of infection. Since most babies are now born in hospitals rather than at home, birth emergencies such as placenta previa and transverse delivery no longer take such a toll in injury to mothers and infants. Neonatal emergencies, such as hypoglycemia and tetany, are no longer such threats to newborn infants. The modern hospital can offer immediate intervention when such emergencies arise. Good prenatal care for all pregnant women could further reduce the incidence of birth accidents and injuries.

VII

Postnatal Causes of Mental Retardation

The postnatal period refers to any time following six weeks of age. There are a number of causes for brain damage occurring during this period, some of which are difficult to identify. Many of the same threats which can cause brain damage and mental retardation during the prenatal and neonatal periods can also produce damage during the postnatal period. These include infections of the central nervous system (brain and spinal cord), injuries, poisons, anoxia and endocrine (glandular) disorders. Less common contributors are tumors, uncontrolled severe convulsions and allergic reactions. It is often difficult for a physician to make an accurate diagnosis because of the fact that various problems other than brain damage may cause a child with average intelligence to function at a retarded level. Emotional problems and maternal and cultural deprivation can all cause a normal child to appear to be mentally retarded.

The central nervous system may become infected by a number of organisms, ranging in size from the viruses, which are invisible even under the microscope, to the bacteria, which are microscopic, and the fungi and other parasites, which are visible to the naked eye. These organisms can enter the brain by several routes, one being the bloodstream. For example, some part of the body becomes infected (usually the lungs), and thus the organism enters the bloodstream, which carries it to the brain. Before the advent of antibiotics, severe infections of the sinuses and of the ears sometimes ate through the bony barrier of the skull and infected the brain.

Usually the organisms which enter and infect the brain itself are viruses. A virus infection of the brain is called *encephalitis,* and it is very dangerous, since viruses can actually destroy brain cells. Occasionally, even the poliomyelitis virus, as well as that of mumps and regular measles, may invade the central nervous system, causing encephalitis. The acute symptoms of encephalitis are headache, seizures and lethargy; the residual effects of the disease are mental retardation, cerebral palsy, seizures and behavior problems. One type of encephalitis has been called sleeping sickness because of the extreme lethargy of the victims. There are still no drugs that are effective in treating viral infections, so there is no treatment other than rest.

Bacteria are somewhat larger than viruses, and they do not usually invade the brain itself, but they do attack the meninges (tissue covering the brain). Such an infection is called purulent meningitis. Any number of common bacterial agents can cause this disease. Children with meningitis are acutely ill and are always considered medical emergencies. Fever, headache and a stiff neck and back are common early symptoms. Convulsions may occur during meningitis, and they can have serious consequences. Fortunately, bacterial infections are sensitive to antibiotics, and most children can survive with adequate therapy. In 10 to 20 percent of the cases, however, there is residual brain damage, resulting in mental retardation, convulsions, learning disorders or deafness.

Other microscopic organisms that can cause mental retardation if they infect the central nervous system are rickettsiae, protozoans and fungi, but such infections are relatively rare in the United States. Tuberculosis, which can cause mental retardation if it infects the brain, is not a serious cause of mental retardation in this country, since there now are specific drugs to treat this disease. It is possible for the tuberculosis organism to enter the central nervous system after infecting the lungs; the victim contracts the infection from some person with whom he is in close contact. The symptoms of such a brain infection are fever, vomiting and convulsions. Diagnosis can be made by examination of the cerebrospinal fluid, the fluid which bathes the brain and spinal cord. This fluid is obtained for examination by a procedure, known as a spinal puncture, in which a needle is inserted into the spinal canal and fluid drawn off. If the infection is found to be tuberculous, treatment with appropriate drugs is begun. Recovery is dependent upon the extent of the tuberculosis invasion present at the time when therapy is initiated. Widespread skin testing for tuberculosis is especially important in the elimination of tuberculous infections. When tuberculosis is identified and treated in its early stages, the spread of the organism to the central nervous system is prevented.

Malnutrition has a relationship to infections in that children who suffer from prolonged nutritional deprivation become weakened and are not able to withstand as well as the average child the organisms to which they are exposed. These children, who are thus predisposed to infection, are more likely to contract the type of infection which could cause brain damage.

There is some question as to whether or not severe malnutrition in itself causes mental retardation. Evidence indicates that older children seem to be able to withstand caloric deprivation, but recent studies have led researchers to believe that infants suffering from severe malnutrition develop mental retardation. Doctors have known for many years that certain specific deficiencies cause certain illnesses. Pellagra is such a disorder; it results from an insufficient intake of vitamin B_5. Pellagra causes mental retardation, but, fortunately, it is practically nonexistent in the United States today. Also, deficiency of vitamin B_6 in infants, causes convulsions and mental retardation.

Recently, the use of megavitamin therapy (huge dosage of vitamins) has been advocated by some for treatment of mentally retarded persons. In certain specific disorders, such as methylmalonicaciduria (inability of the body to use vitamin B_{12}), very large doses of certain specific vitamins are indeed required for survival. However, the theory that certain retarded children need enormous amounts of vitamins and minerals to flush the impurities from their bodies has not been proven scientifically, and it has been shown that such dosages are not effective in reversing mental retardation. It is unfortunate that some people have spent large sums of money for such treatment for their children in the hope that their mental retardation could be reversed.

The lack of certain substances in the diet can indirectly cause mental retardation. For many years it has been known that there is an association between the lack of iodine in the diet and goiter, with resulting hypothyroidism and mental retardation. Fortunately, in many countries today, hypothyroidism due to lack of iodine in the diet is very rare because of the use of iodized salt. Iodized salt may be something that we all take for granted, but it is very important in areas where there is an inadequate amount of iodine in the water. The thyroid gland cannot function without a supply of iodine, and without thyroid hormone a person becomes mentally retarded because it is necessary for proper brain cell metabolism.

Hypothyroidism can also be caused by a sluggish thyroid gland which fails to provide the necessary amount of thyroid hormone. In some cases, it is almost nonfunctioning. The person who is hypothyroid is lethargic, short and pudgy, has coarse facial features, sparse hair, dry skin, chronic constipation and mental retardation. Early diagnosis is very important, since the symptoms can be reversed and the mental retardation prevented if treatment is begun promptly. Once the disorder has advanced to the point where the brain tissue is damaged, however, treatment will alleviate the physical symptoms but cannot reverse the mental retardation. This disorder can usually be diagnosed by the visible symptoms, and laboratory tests can confirm the diagnosis. Treatment consists of the administration of thyroid extract, which is dramatically effective in alleviating the symptoms and preventing mental retardation if begun in time.

Since the occurrence of mental retardation can be prevented by early diagnosis, the importance of regular medical checkups in childhood must be emphasized. Even today, approximately one out of every hundred persons in institutions for the mentally retarded suffers from hypothyroidism. (There are no other major endocrine causes of mental retardation known at this time.)

The following story of Maria demonstrates the tragedy of untreated hypothyroidism. Maria was first diagnosed properly when she was seen by the doctor at a clinic associated with a school for mentally retarded children. Eleven years old, she was thirty-two inches tall and weighed thirty pounds. Her skin was very dry, her hair was sparse and dry, and she was chronically constipated. Her legs were swollen as a result of fluid retention. She had no speech and she had a very dull appearance. The doctor made the diagnosis of cretinism, and she was put on a dosage of one-half grain of thyroid daily. This dosage was gradually increased to two grains daily. When Maria was seen at the clinic six months later, she had grown nearly four inches. She was no longer retaining fluid in her tissues, her skin and hair appeared healthy, and she looked bright-eyed and alert. She was still mentally retarded and had little speech, but her dramatic improvement continued. At the end of a year, she had grown six inches. Unfortunately, Maria will always be mentally retarded. If she had been diagnosed and treated within the first three months of life, the mental retardation could have been avoided.

The following case history shows the value of early treatment in cases of hypothyroidism. S.C. was first seen by a doctor at the age of two months because of lethargy, puffy eyelids, protuberant abdomen and a history of jaundice.

She had been of normal weight when she was born, but her mother had noted that she had become lethargic and had been sleeping long periods between feedings. There was no history of constipation, which is usually a symptom of hypothyroidism, although she exhibited all the classic signs of the disorder. She was a dull, sleepy infant with dry, coarse skin, large protruding tongue, bulging abdomen, and large, puffy legs (the result of fluid retention in the tissues).

Laboratory tests indicated a significant absence of thyroid function. She was immediately started on one-eighth grain of thyroid daily. This dosage was doubled every two weeks until a full two grains of thyroid were being administered daily. Her developmental status began to improve rapidly. By one year of age, she was testing within normal limits on the Gesell developmental scales. Her last intelligence quotient at six years of age was 101. At present, she is taking four grains of thyroid daily. She is a junior in high school, and is of average height and weight.

Another serious problem is iron deficiency. This does not in itself cause mental retardation, but the resulting anemia predisposes infants to infection, which, as mentioned before, can cause damage to the brain.

A problem on the increase today in all developed countries is that of injury caused by automobile accidents. Nature has provided more protection for the brain—in the form of the skull—than for any other part of the body. The skull can withstand many minor injuries without permanent damage to the brain, but it is no match for the heavy glass and metal of the modern automobile.

Concussion usually occurs when there is a sudden jarring of the head which causes the capillaries in the brain to rupture. This causes bleeding into the surface of the brain. When a concussion is slight, as in a minor skull fracture, only a week or two of rest may be required for full recovery. A person suffering a brain injury may become nauseated and incoherent, and may lose consciousness. When a child exhibits these symptoms of injury to the brain, the head is X-rayed to rule out the possibility of a depressed skull fracture. In the case of a minor skull fracture or a concussion, the only treatment is bed rest; but with a depressed skull fracture, in which a portion of the skull is pushed down into the brain, the depressed bit of bone must be removed surgically. In such cases, recovery depends upon the extent of the injury. If there has been actual destruction of brain tissue, permanent damage may result.

In serious injuries to the head, there is always the danger of the development of *subdural hematoma*. This occurs when an artery of the brain has been damaged and is releasing blood into the subdural space between the dura (tough, outer membrane covering the brain) and the brain itself. The accumulation of blood can compress the brain, so prompt surgery is necessary to release the pressure and prevent permanent damage.

Injury to the brain does not necessarily result in mental retardation; it depends upon the portion of the brain involved. Damage to the part of the brain governing muscular movement can cause various types of muscular disorders, such as cerebral palsy, without affecting mental ability. The thinking parts of the brain are predominantly in the outer portions, commonly called the cerebral cortex or the gray matter. When these portions of the brain are damaged, mental retardation does result.

A problem which is increasingly being brought to the attention of pediatricians is that of the "battered child," the child who has suffered injury at the hands of an adult, usually his parents or a baby-sitter. Such injury is generally inflicted in a fit of anger. The child is usually brought to the hospital with unexplained bone fractures or with a history of vomiting, enlarging head, failing vision and convulsions. Such children are often found to be suffering from chronic subdural hematomas as a result of frequent blows to the head. Surgery is required in such cases to remove the massive blood clots from the brain. Several such children who are mentally retarded as a result of repeated cerebral injury have been seen at the Mental Retardation Clinic at Childrens Hospital in Los Angeles.

In most states the law requires that the physician report suspected cases of battered children to the police.

In such cases, until the competency of the parents has been established the child is usually released to other relatives. If the parents are found guilty, they may be prosecuted and the child put in foster care.

Another postnatal cause of mental retardation is poisoning. Of course all poisons are especially dangerous to young children, and in case of emergency, parents should be aware of the nearest poison center. Lead poisoning is the worst offender as far as mental retardation is concerned. This insidious type of poisoning does not cause an immediate problem; it usually accumulates in the child's system, without the parents being aware of the exposure until the child exhibits symptoms of headache, vomiting and convulsions. The exposure to lead usually comes from old paint. Although most paint manufactured today does not contain lead, in the past nearly all paint did. Leaded paint was even used on baby toys and furniture; thus every time a baby sucked a painted toy or chewed a crib rail, he ingested lead. Even today, most cases of lead poisoning are the result of children chewing and eating paint from window sills and woodwork in old houses. This is especially true in the East, where the homes are older. Lead poisoning can also be caused by the inhalation of battery fumes. And in recent years the smog in our cities has added to the problem. Ethyl gasoline contains a considerable amount of lead. The amount of lead in the systems of most people is rising, and most city dwellers have higher lead levels than do people in rural areas. When a dangerously high level of lead becomes chronic in the system, it is deposited in various tissues and organs, including the brain. These deposits interfere with the brain-cell metabolism, and the resulting mental retardation is usually severe. In other words, when the brain cannot secure the necessary nourishment, its cells are damaged and mental retardation occurs.

At present, treatment for lead poisoning is available

in the form of an injectable chemical which combines with the lead in the body, and is then excreted in the urine. Recently, screening tests have been devised to detect elevated lead levels in the body before the poisoning has reached a serious stage. Research is being conducted to determine how practical mass screening will be in preventing lead poisoning.

Anoxia and resultant brain damage can occur whenever a person is denied oxygen. Any person who does not breathe for four minutes runs the risk of suffering brain damage. Accidental suffocation can be caused by near drowning, by plastic bags covering the heads of small children, or by strangulation. The same complications result from cardiac arrest (temporary stopping of the heart) because of the lack of oxygenated blood circulating through the brain, and from carbon monoxide poisoning, in which the hemoglobin in the blood is prevented from carrying oxygen to the brain.

Disorders involving the process of metabolism account for about 5 percent of all retardation. These diseases are sometimes called inborn errors of metabolism, as they are usually genetic diseases determined at the time of conception. Many of these diseases can now be diagnosed and some can be treated. Research is progressing rapidly in this area. Phenylketonuria is one such disease which can now be diagnosed and treated, and mental retardation prevented. Galactosemia is another such disease, but it is rare (one in every forty thousand births), so testing is not done on a large scale at the present time. It would be simple and inexpensive to test all babies for this disease at birth, and in the long run, it would be worthwhile in preventing the tragedy and expense of mental retardation in those children who are affected.

Maple syrup urine disease, hyperglycinemia, methylmalonicaciduria and histidinemia are four more metabolic diseases which cause mental retardation but which are now diagnosable and treatable. Although doctors have not learned to cure these diseases, they have learned to control them through diet. There is much to be learned in this field (for example, doctors do not yet know exactly how insulin works in controlling diabetes). The study of exactly which enzymes break down the various food elements is complicated, but as medical research continues in this area, it is inevitable that other metabolic diseases will be recognized and treatments devised.

Mental retardation can also be caused during the postnatal period by brain tumors, which damage brain tissue as they expand. They are rare in children, however, and with modern surgical techniques, doctors are increasingly able to successfully treat such disorders.

Cerebrovascular accidents (strokes) are also very uncommon in childhood, but do occur occasionally, and they can cause brain damage.

There are also certain degenerative disorders of the central nervous system which can cause mental retardation. These disorders are not well classified as yet, and they are even less well understood. Tay-Sachs Disease is one such disorder. This insidious, genetic defect strikes one in every 3,600 infants whose parents descended from Ashkenazi Jews, who settled in Eastern Europe around A.D. 700. Judaism prohibited the Jews from marrying Gentiles, and until 1880, nearly all Eastern European countries had strict laws prohibiting Christian and Jewish intermarriage. The interfamily marriage which took place in the Jewish ghettos brought on Tay-Sachs Disease, because this disorder is caused by a recessive genetic defect in which an enzyme, hexosaminidase A, is missing. When two carriers of the disease marry, one in four of their offspring will have the disease and two in four will be carriers. In this disease, which was first described by Dr. Warren Tay and Dr. Bernard Sachs in 1880, the victim appears normal at birth, but usually around the age of four to eight months he begins to lose vitality. He degenerates progressively with convulsions, becoming blind, helpless and mentally retarded. One of the early symptoms is a cherry-red spot in the eye. It is only visible upon examination with an ophthalmoscope, but it can confirm a diagnosis of Tay-Sachs Disease. It is caused by a change in the retina of the eye, in which the rods and cones which are the receptors of visual stimuli degenerate and expose the capillary bed behind them, causing the spot and also bringing on blindness. Death is inevitable and usually occurs within three to five years. Dr. Michael Kaback has recently devised a blood test which has proven to be 100 percent accurate in identifying Tay-Sachs Disease carriers. The disease can also be detected in utero by amniocentesis. This dramatic breakthrough has the potential of eradicating Tay-Sachs Disease. In dollars and cents, this will mean a saving to the state of $100,000 to $200,000 for each Tay-Sachs victim, since these children are nearly always put in the state institutions because of the severity of the disease. (At the present time in California, there are five to ten Tay-Sachs patients in state institutions at all times.) Beyond the reduction in cost, there is the immeasurable benefit of preventing human suffering and tragedy in affected families.

A patient, B.D., was referred to the author at the age of nine months because his pediatrician suspected that he had Tay-Sachs Disease but lacked the laboratory facilities necessary to verify the diagnosis.

The parents were both of Jewish ancestry, but there was no history of mental retardation on either side of the family. There was one three-year-old normal brother. B.D.

had had a normal delivery and had developed normally until he began to have seizures at five months of age. He had been given a number of anti-convulsant medications, but none of them had been effective in controlling the seizures. His parents reported that prior to the onset of seizures the baby had been smiling, feeding well, and was able to roll over, but after the onset of seizures he had become apathetic, smiled less often and seemed irritable.

The physical examination revealed a well-developed, well-nourished nine-month-old baby, who appeared outwardly normal, but who was significantly retarded mentally. He had poor head control and he did not reach for and grasp articles. He had some increased spasticity and clonus (repetitive movement of the foot in response to stimulation of the sole with a hard object), and his knee and ankle jerks were hyperactive. The most significant symptom was the cherry-red spot which the doctor noted on examination of the eye. The diagnosis of Tay-Sachs Disease was confirmed by the laboratory report. The baby's blood contained no hexosaminidase A activity.

Since there is no treatment for Tay-Sachs Disease, B.D. degenerated progressively and died at the age of two years. The mother has had no more pregnancies. She was counseled to have amniocentesis should she become pregnant again.

Allergic reactions can also cause mental retardation in rare cases. For example, a child may have an allergic reaction to a specific vaccine, such as smallpox or rabies. In such cases, the patient will have encephalitis-like symptoms of lethargy and convulsions. Such reactions are very rare, but when they do happen they can cause mental retardation, and unfortunately, there is no treatment at the present time.

Psychiatric factors in the field of mental retardation have been thoroughly studied. It is not uncommon for children who are mentally retarded to develop some abnormal behavior patterns which seem psychiatric in nature. Some retarded children become mute, play for long periods alone and are seldom affectionate. They often twirl and play with spinning objects, such as wheels, balls, coins and tops. Some of them walk only on their toes. In fact, many times it is difficult to tell whether such children are truly retarded or whether their problem is purely emotional or both. These children are typically called autistic. Autism is more likely to afflict children who were premature and in some children with convulsive disorders, but it can occur in children of normal intelligence. It is interesting that about 80 to 90 percent of autistic children are boys, and the condition seldom appears twice in the same family. There is much research going on in this field at present, and there is even a national society for the study of autistic children. To date, however, the outlook for these children is poor.

One disorder which used to cause mental retardation can now be treated surgically to prevent brain damage. Called *craniosynostosis,* this is a condition in which the fissures of the skull are fused together at birth. Nearly all infants have a fontanel (soft spot at the top of the head) at birth and during the first year of life. The reason for this is that the bones of the skull have open fissures or sutures between them which enable the infant's head to contract during the birth process. During the first year, it expands to cover the very rapidly growing brain. Usually by the time the child reaches the age of one or two years, the fissures of the skull have joined together around the brain. In craniosynostosis, however, these sutures have already fused by the time the baby is born. In such cases, the skull cannot expand as the child's brain grows, resulting in brain damage and mental retardation. It is unusual for all of the sutures to be fused at birth, but it does happen occasionally. When only one or two of the sutures are fused, the head expands only where there are open fissures, producing an abnormally shaped head. Sagittal synostosis (fusion of the sagittal fissure) is the most common form of this disorder. The sagittal suture is the central fissure which extends along the crown of the head from front to back. When the sagittal suture is fused, the skull cannot broaden; therefore it expands where it can, becoming disproportionately long from forehead to back, in comparison with its width. Coronal synostosis involves the coronal sutures which cross the head from ear to ear. When these sutures are fused, the head becomes broad and high but cannot expand from front to back. There are other variations of this disorder. Sometimes there is only a partial coronal involvement. The right coronal suture may be fused, while the left is normal. In such a case, the right side of the forehead would be small and the left side would bulge. In the past, children with this disorder became retarded because their brains could not expand properly as they grew. With modern surgery, the fused sutures can be opened so that the brain of the affected child can develop normally.

The following case history of Patty B. was reported by Betty Graliker, chief counselor at the Child Development Clinic at Childrens Hospital in Los Angeles. This case illustrates the manner in which an average American family of modest income was suddenly faced with a severe medical problem, and how the parents reacted initially and how they themselves grew as they lived with it.

Patty was the youngest of four children. She had a sister twelve years older than herself and two brothers ten and seven years older.

Patty was first seen at Childrens Hospital at the age

of eighteen days. She was referred by her family physician because she had been born with webbing of all her fingers and toes, a cleft palate, and premature closure of the cranial sutures. The baby's general condition was good except for the marked brachycephaly (misshapen head, short from front to back) due to coronal synostosis. The infant was diagnosed as having Apert's Syndrome, the cause of which is not known. In Patty's case, her mother had had hepatitis during the first three months of the pregnancy. There was no family history of congenital defects and one of the first comments of her father was, "We never had anything like this in our family."

A craniectomy (removal of a portion of the skull on either side of the affected suture to allow the brain to grow normally) was performed immediately. Although the surgery was successful, Patty's head did not assume a normal shape at once. It took several years for this to happen. Most of the treatment of the baby was on an outpatient basis, and the father often accompanied his wife when she brought the baby to the hospital, since he worked a night shift. The parents were sensitive about the baby's appearance, and always concealed her face in public. Later her mother commented, "At first I didn't want anyone to see her." The parents also worried that Patty would be mentally retarded. Her father especially had difficulty in accepting the child, and wanted to know, "What will people think of her . . . what will they think of me for having such a child? What do people do with such children? Do they put them in homes?" Patty's mother had some doubts, too, but she wanted to do what was right for the family, and she felt the child could fit into their home.

Patty's medical care was coordinated by the Child Development Clinic and the parents relied on the clinic staff for counseling. Patty received regular physical examinations and developmental testing. At the age of five years, her IQ was 65, but with each test she showed gradual improvement, and her parents were advised to take one step at a time, rather than trying to plan her whole future. The social worker was especially helpful to the mother in providing moral support and interpreting the medical program, and in discussing with her the various problems as they arose.

As time went on, Patty began to develop a pleasing personality, and she continued to show improvement. Her mother always took special care to dress her attractively, and started taking her out in public when she was about two years old. When she was two and a half, her mother began taking her to the church nursery on Sundays. Her father still did not feel completely comfortable taking her out in public, and he worried about the reception she would have when the family visited his parents in another state. He was very relieved when they accepted and loved her as they did the other children. Mr. B. finally also felt comfortable in taking Patty out with him in public.

When she was four years old, Patty began attending a class sponsored by the Exceptional Children's Foundation. The group met daily. When she was five years old, her parents entered her in a regular kindergarten. They were not certain that their decision was correct, and felt that perhaps she should go to a kindergarten for physically handicapped children. Her father was especially reluctant, fearing that the other children might make fun of her, but the school principal felt that the staff could handle the situation. During that year, Patty started a series of operations on her hands. It took two years to complete the operations, but the results were very good, and now she has almost normal use of her hands.

The wisdom of sending her to regular kindergarten was borne out by the comments of her teacher.

"Patty came to kindergarten as any normal child. She

did not expect favors and babying. She tried and enjoyed everything the others in the group did. The thing that gave her the most trouble was opening her milk carton. But in a few weeks, she was able to do that. At first, standing in line bothered her because of her poor balance (kindergartners do push in line occasionally); she never said anything, but if I was near her, she would steady herself on me.

"We often play circle games and I have never seen a child refuse to hold hands with Patty.

"I don't know that any child in the room knew Patty before school started, and after discussing it in the office with the nurse and secretary, I decided before school started that I would do nothing formal in the way of 'preparing' them for Patty or 'explaining her to them,' for, after all, they were just a bunch of scared little beginners themselves. Of course they noticed her hands, but the only time they were actually discussed was when she was absent before Christmas for her surgery, and when I told them she was going to have her hands operated on, one little girl said, 'So she can do like this?' and spread her fingers flat. That seemed to satisfy them all and no more questions were asked. The group was always happy to hear that she was progressing well and were glad to have her back. Now we are anxious for her to come back from the second operation.

"Her speech has been her greatest improvement. It was about November that I realized that she was speaking more clearly. She had learned last year to recognize her own name and surprised me by naming the letters as I wrote them on her paint paper.

"Patty has done something special with this group of children just by being one of them. They have accepted her so completely that I hope their attitude will stay with them whenever they are in contact with someone who is not as fortunate as they."

The family continued to live from day to day, not looking too far ahead. The parents set limited goals for Patty. They did all in their power to make her socially acceptable, correcting her handicaps through surgery and speech therapy. As they lived with this problem the parents grew in insight and maturity. At one point, Mr. B. said, "We are just as happy as we can be with her. She gets along fine in the family. We take her everywhere. You know, at first, you kind of feel funny about a child like that . . . kind of ashamed, but you finally get over that."

After kindergarten, Patty went to a school for physically handicapped children. Her academic achievements have not been outstanding, but she has continued to improve. Her last IQ score was 76. She recently graduated from high school. She has been referred to a vocational rehabilitation center where she can learn a skill so that she will be employable.

Patty's parents were fortunate that Mr. B. had very good group health insurance where he worked. His insurance paid for 80 percent of the medical costs for Patty. The rest was paid for by the Crippled Children's Service, which is supported by federal, state and local taxes, and is available to any child who has a crippling condition. Without this help, the B.'s surely could not have paid for all the medical and surgical costs involved in Patty's care, and Patty might have spent her life in an institution for the retarded, completely helpless; instead, she will be a contributing, independent member of society.

There are other disorders causing mental retardation which are involved with obvious abnormalities in the size and shape of the head. One of these is *hydrocephalus*. The term literally means water on the brain, and afflicted children have exceptionally large heads. There are a number of causes for this condition, not all of which are actually associated with excessive fluid within the skull. Some babies just naturally have rather large heads, which are perfectly normal. However, abnormal enlargement of the skull and brain damage can be caused by such disorders as brain tumors and subdural hematomas (blood clots). As a tumor or subdural hematoma grows, the brain is damaged and the skull enlarges to accommodate it.

Blockage of the cerebrospinal fluid can also cause brain damage and enlargement of the skull. In order to understand this disorder, one should know how the cerebrospinal fluid circulates through the brain and spinal canal. In the central part of the brain is an area called the choroid plexus where the cerebrospinal fluid is manufactured. Above and below the choroid plexus, there are cavities (ventricles). As the cerebrospinal fluid is produced, it circulates up through the ventricles and down to the base of the brain where it flows up the outside of the brain. It is thought by some that a large portion of it is absorbed here by the gray matter or the cortex. It also flows down through the spinal canal, which is an extension of the brain. Although doctors do not know the exact purpose of the cerebrospinal fluid, they do know it is carried to all parts of the brain. Some say the purpose is to give the brain a protective cushion of fluid. Others feel the fluid may be a source of energy for the brain, and another theory is that it may help remove metabolic waste material.

Whatever its purpose, if for any reason the flow of this fluid is obstructed, it builds up in the ventricles of the brain, eventually causing the gray matter to atrophy from the pressure, and causing the skull to enlarge. There are two main forms of hydrocephalus: obstructive and communicating.

In obstructive hydrocephalus, the canal carrying the cerebrospinal fluid becomes blocked near the base of the brain, causing the fluid to collect in the ventricles. The cause of this disorder is usually present at birth, but it can also be caused by meningitis, brain tumor or birth injury due to a breech delivery. This form of the disease can be diagnosed by injecting a dye through the fontanel and into a ventricle of the brain, and then performing a spinal tap. If there is no obstruction, the dyed fluid should circulate to the site of the spinal tap within a few minutes. If, however, no fluid containing dye is obtained in the tap, the diagnosis of obstructive hydrocephalus can be made. The disorder can be treated surgically by connecting a small tube above and below the obstruction so that it is by-passed. Such a by-pass can be performed wherever an obstruction may occur.

In the communicating form of hydrocephalus, there is no obstruction, but when the fluid reaches the cortex, or gray matter, it is thought that it is not properly absorbed, and as in the obstructive form of the disease, it eventually collects in the ventricles of the brain. The treatment involves the placing of a small tube leading from one of the ventricles of the brain to the large vessel leading to the heart (the superior vena cava); through the tube the excess fluid is drained away into the bloodstream. This procedure is called a ventriculocardiac shunt. When it was first tried, a problem was encountered in that the blood from the heart was under more pressure than was the cerebrospinal fluid, thereby causing the blood to flow into the tube instead of the fluid flowing into the blood vessel. A special valve was invented to fit into the end of the tube and prevent the flow of blood into it, making this form of treatment practicable. (Holter, the engineer who invented the valve, was the father of a hydrocephalic child.) One might suppose that when the fluid is not absorbed by the gray matter and is drained away in this manner, some brain damage might result. This has not proven to be true. Doctors know mental retardation can be prevented by this procedure, but they do not know exactly why.

Hydrocephalus can also be caused by a congenital disorder involving the spine in which there is a distortion or defect in alignment of the spinal column, with the vertebrae (bones surrounding the spinal cord) actually forming a curve or loop. Attached to this spinal derangement is a pouch of cerebrospinal fluid and spongy tissue. This pouch is called a *meningomyelocele*, or more commonly the disorder is known as *spina bifida*. Usually, some of the cerebrospinal fluid which collects at the site of the defect drains off through its surface. This tissue can be removed surgically, and there are now some efforts being made to correct the spinal defect as well. Occasionally, following surgery for this condition, the fluid which was escaping through the meningomyelocele is blocked and hydrocephalus results, but spina bifida is not always accompanied by hydrocephalus. The spinal nerves are usually damaged by the defect, resulting in paraplegia (paralysis of the lower limbs), loss of bladder and rectal control, and loss of sensation in the lower extremities. The primary problem is the spinal defect and the damage to the spinal nerves. The hydrocephalus which is caused by spina bifida can also be treated by the use of the ventriculocardiac shunt, but because of the added problem of the spinal defect the prognosis is usually poor for such patients.

In concluding this discussion of postnatal causes of mental retardation, the relationship between poverty and mental retardation cannot be escaped. In fact, poverty may be a leading cause of mental retardation. Psychologists and physicians in the field of mental retardation have known for some time that certain groups of children appear to have a high incidence of mental retardation. For example, a disproportionate number of retarded children have come from poor families and minority groups. The child born to a poorly educated, low-income family living in a slum environment is predestined to have a lower intelligence than the child born and raised in a middle- or upper-class environment.

Poverty can affect a child before he is born. His mother may suffer malnutrition during the pregnancy. She will probably not have had rubella immunization. It is very likely that she will have had no prenatal care. Indeed, the President's Committee on Mental Retardation reported in 1968 that 45 percent of all women having babies in public hospitals had had no prenatal care, causing added risks to both themselves and their babies. It may be discovered too late that the mother has produced a child damaged by Rh factor blood incompatibility. She may be suffering from toxemia by the time she finally seeks medical help, or she may have tried to induce an abortion during the pregnancy and succeeded only in damaging the child. The child's delivery may be made hazardous by a lack of foreknowledge about such abnormal conditions as a very large baby, an abnormal position of the fetus and placenta previa. The child has triple the chances of a middle-class child of being born prematurely, and prematurity itself puts the baby at greater risk. Neurological and physical disorders are 75 percent more frequent among premature babies than among full-term ones.

The infant begins his social and intellectual growth immediately after birth. In a deprived environment he is again at a greater risk than a child in a higher socioeconomic group. Because of a poor diet, his resistance to disease and infection may be low. The mother may have to go to work almost immediately, leaving the infant in the care of an older sister, or perhaps with little care at all. Left alone in a crib in drab, unstimulating surroundings, he will not learn to interact with people, as will a child who is cuddled, played with and talked to. Without receiving warmth and love, he will probably be unable to form close relationships later. His language development will be delayed, as he must hear sounds and words on which to pattern his own speech. This deficiency can, of course, occur in any family regardless of socioeconomic status, but it is more likely to occur when the parents must use all their energy just earning the necessities of life. In such circumstances there is little time left for giving extra attention to a baby. By the time the slum child reaches school age, he is usually completely unprepared to learn to read and write and count. Without the experience or ability to learn these new skills, such a child is apt to fall further and further behind and eventually drop out of school. In the slums, children also face a risk of infection through rat bite. This is a serious problem which affects many children each year. According to the National Advisory Commission on Civil Disorders, it is estimated that in 1965 there were more than 14,000 cases of rat bite in the United States, mostly in deprived neighborhoods. They are also more likely to be exposed to lead poisoning from ingesting paint. Modern paint does not contain lead, but old, deteriorating buildings are apt to have peeling paint containing this deadly substance.

Lack of knowledge of birth control methods compounds the problems for the poor. It has long been possible for those who can afford it to avail themselves of birth control devices, and even to have abortions under safe, sanitary conditions. This has not been the case for the poor. Without money for visits to the doctor and birth control pills or devices, the women living in poverty may bear one child after another, whom they cannot properly feed or care for. Or, in desperation, they may seek abortions from people with no medical training.

Thus the dreadful cycle continues: poverty, malnutrition, inadequate and unsanitary living conditions, illness and mental retardation. In 1967 the late Whitney Young, then executive director of the National Urban League, said that the poverty world of the Blacks, Mexican laborers, American Indians, Puerto Rican immigrants and poor whites is "the breeding ground of as much as half of our mentally retarded people, the dull-eyed children, the juvenile delinquents, the dropouts and socially unadaptable youngsters, who drive teachers, lawmakers and governments to despair!"

The recent decision of the Supreme Court legalizing abortions, along with the current emphasis on birth control and family planning, should help alleviate this situation, but there is still a long way to go. A National Health Insurance plan should be established by the federal government, making good health the right of every citizen, and not just the privilege of those who can afford medical care.

There should be good prenatal care and food supplements for all pregnant women. No unborn child should be doomed to be brain-damaged because his mother could not afford to go to the doctor during her pregnancy. There should be a national school-lunch program so that children in poverty areas could have good, nutritious lunches at school. It is inexcusable that there should be hungry children in this wealthy country. And the government should do more in the way of educating the public regarding the importance of good prenatal care for mothers and of immunizations for all babies. How many women of the child-bearing age know that three-day measles can permanently damage an unborn child? How many women in the child-bearing years even know whether or not they have ever had three-day measles? How many realize the importance of finding out whether or not they are immune to this disease and of getting immunized if they are not? How many women realize that good prenatal care can, in many cases, avert the birth of a brain-damaged child? What woman would not want to avail herself of good health care if she knew these things? Five million dollars a year spent in advertising good health care would pay off in a significant reduction in the birth of brain-damaged and retarded children.

VIII
Down's Syndrome

Most people have heard the term "Mongolism" used at one time or another, but relatively few have an adequate understanding of this condition, a chromosome disorder in which a number of physical abnormalities as well as mental retardation are present. It is hoped that the information given here will help the reader to better understand this largest single, easily identifiable group of mentally retarded individuals.

Professionals in the field of retardation now refer to this disorder as Down's syndrome, or D.S.

Down's syndrome is named in honor of Dr. John Langdon-Down, who identified it. In 1886, he reported that certain individuals had a number of symptoms in common, including slanting, Oriental-appearing eyes, shortness of stature, stubby hands, flattened nasal bridges, small mouths with drooping corners, protruding tongues, white speckled irises of the eyes, and mental retardation. Dr. Down mistakenly assumed that all such persons were severely retarded, and labeled them Mongolian idiots because of their Oriental appearance and their supposed low intelligence. Unfortunately, this term came into general use, with many people assuming that all such individuals were indeed hopelessly retarded, and that perhaps they were somehow descended from the Mongolian race. It is now known that this condition is caused by an extra no. 21 chromosome in each cell of the body, making a total of 47 chromosomes for the D.S. individual, rather than the normal complement of 46. We now know also that rarely does this disorder occur in true Mongolians, and contrary to Dr. Down's supposition that all such persons are idiots, the disorder occurs in all degrees of severity, sometimes causing only mild retardation.

D.S. occurs in approximately one in every 700 births. It is estimated that 65,000 D.S. individuals live in the United States alone. Most of this group requires supervised care, accounting for about 10 percent of all retarded persons receiving residential care outside their homes.

Because of the distinguishing characteristics, the diagnosis can easily be made in 90 to 95 percent of cases. Actually, some fifty known characteristics are associated with D.S. All of these characteristics do not necessarily occur in each person with D.S., and occasionally an individual with normal intelligence exhibits several of them. Usually, however, most of them are present in the true D.S. person, and unfortunately, nearly all such individuals suffer mental retardation. Although the diagnosis is usually easily made, occasionally there are cases where the typical signs, such as slanting eyes and protruding tongue, are minimal or nearly absent, and even the most experienced clinician may be faced with a difficult task in making a correct diagnosis. Such "borderline" cases can only be diagnosed accurately by chromosomal study. This relatively new field of study is called *cytogenetics*.

When the technique of chromosome counting first became available, it was very expensive and time-consuming. It usually took from six to eight weeks for results to be obtained; therefore, cytogenetic studies were recommended only in carefully selected cases—usually young mothers whose firstborn children had had D.S. In such cases it was felt likely that the D.S. was of a hereditary type and cytogenetic studies were considered indispensable for good genetic counseling. Advancements have been made in this technique, and it has become less expensive. Cytogeneticists can now isolate the chromosomes in a sample of blood cells, examine them for abnormalities in formation and count them, and then have the results in one or two weeks. They have found that there are at least fourteen types of chromosomal abnormalities which can cause this disorder, so it is referred to as the D.S. complex. All of these abnormalities result in an extra no. 21 chromosome, which is typical of D.S.

Some forms of D.S. are hereditary, while others are merely accidental mutations, so it is important to establish the type of defect in order that families may receive proper genetic counseling. This makes cytogenetic studies very important, and now that the technique has been simplified they are performed on all retarded persons who have any of the D.S. symptoms. If a child is found to have a hereditary form of D.S., the parents themselves are advised to have cytogenetic studies done on them to determine which of them is the carrier of the defect so that genetic counseling can be given to the appropriate relatives. Such a couple may decide against having other children of their own. They would certainly be advised to have amniocentesis if another pregnancy did occur, since D.S. can be detected in utero. If the fetus is found to have D.S., the parents may decide that an abortion would be preferable to bringing another mentally retarded child into the world. If the cytogenetic study finds that the D.S. is not of a hereditary form, the parents can be reassured that they are not a high-risk couple but there would be on the average a 1 to 2 percent risk of a second-born D.S. child. For this reason, many of these parents would also elect to have amniocentesis with all subsequent pregnancies.

Since some of the chromosomal abnormalities which cause D.S. are very rare and complex, only the most common forms will be discussed here. One form of D.S. which has puzzled doctors in the past has recently been identified and explained.

Within the past five years a number of cases have been reported in medical literature of persons who supposedly had D.S. but had normal intelligence. Through cytogenetic examination, it was found that some of these persons had a combination of normal 46 chromosome cells, in addition to abnormal 47 chromosome cells. In other words, at some point during prenatal mitosis (cell division), a mutation had occurred after a number of normal cells had already reproduced. In such a mutation, instead of one cell dividing into two normal cells with 46 chromosomes each, it had divided into one cell with 45 chromosomes and the other with 47 chromosomes. It is thought that the cells with 45 chromosomes cannot survive because of the loss of so many genes, but the remaining cells, some with 46 chromosomes and some with 47, do survive, and continue to divide normally, eventually forming the new baby. The term applied to such a condition is *mosaicism*.

Mosaics may or may not exhibit the typical characteristics of D.S. The number of symptoms is probably dependent upon the age of the embryo when the mutation occurs. Early misdivision could produce nearly equal numbers of normal and abnormal cells, along with the usual characteristics of D.S., while late misdivision would probably result in a decreased number of abnormal cells, as well as minimal signs of D.S. and probably normal intelligence. Since the mutation which causes mosaicism occurs after fertilization, parents of a mosaic child can be assured that the condition is not hereditary and there is very little chance that a subsequent child would have D.S. or mosaicism.

Although mosaics are usually only mildly retarded and some even have normal intelligence, they can pass D.S. on to their children. In fact, some people do not know they are mosaics until they have a D.S. child and cytogenetic studies reveal the fact that they are mosaics. Therefore, mosaics should be cautioned to have amniocentesis with all pregnancies. Their chances of producing a defective child depend upon the percentage of defective cells in their makeup. For example, a parent in whom 90 percent of the cells have the extra chromosome is more likely to have a D.S. child than a mosaic parent in whom only 10 percent of the cells have 47 chromosomes. Of course, if both parents are mosaics, the risk again increases.

The most common form of D.S. is *trisomy 21*, in which, in place of the no. 21 pair of chromosomes, there is a trisomy (three individual no. 21 chromosomes). All of the cells of individuals having this form of D.S. have 47 chromosomes. This is the noninherited, or sporadic, type of D.S. It occurs in the general population with a frequency of one in seven hundred births. The risk of this type of disorder increases with the aging of the mother. Therefore, younger parents can be reassured that there will be little risk of their having a second child with this form of

CHROMOSOME PAIRS

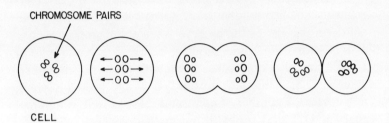

CELL

CELL AND CHROMOSOME DUPLICATION

D.S. According to Dr. Lionel Penrose, who did extensive studies of D.S. in Great Britain, the mother between twenty-two and twenty-four years of age who has a child with this form of D.S. has only one chance in sixteen hundred of having another. Although it is difficult to generalize, and there are factors which sometimes increase this risk, young mothers should not be dissuaded from having other children unless they carry one of the inherited forms of D.S.

On the other hand, it has been found after extensive study that as the mother grows older, her chances of having a child with D.S. are increased considerably. This is explained by the fact that the cells which are destined to form ova are already present in the female body at birth. They remain immature and dormant until puberty, at which time they become mature and are released at monthy intervals for possible fertilization. Therefore, the ova are exposed to a great deal of environmental stress over the years. For example, irradiation, viruses and certain chemicals can damage the chromosomes of the ova. The longer the ova are exposed to damaging influences, the greater is the risk that one of them may become damaged to such an extent that chromosomal changes will take place. When such an ovum is fertilized a D.S. baby may result. It is thought that the ova, rather than the sperm cells, are the defective cells in D.S., because the sperm cells are constantly being formed in the body of the male in such large numbers that the few defective cells are usually unable to compete with the healthy ones in fertilization of the ova. This theory is confirmed by studies failing to show any effect of the age of fathers of children with D.S.

In the cytogenetic study of persons with trisomy 21, at least 10 cells and preferably 21 cells are analyzed to rule out the possibility for mosaicism in the child. Ideally, both parents should also be analyzed in order to rule out the possibility of parental mosaicism. Of course, if either or both of the parents are found to be mosaics, they should receive proper counseling.

The inherited form of D.S. is called *translocation*, and its origin is complicated. Occasionally in the reproduction of normal cells in an embryo, two chromosomes overlap and break at the point of contact, and instead of reuniting in the proper manner, the broken ends join with the wrong chromosome; this usually occurs between the no. 14 and the no. 21 chromosomes. The following is a simplified explanation of the process. Within the nucleus of the normal cell, the pairs of chromosomes are long and intertwined; when the cell prepares to duplicate itself, the chromosomes arrange themselves in rows in preparation for separating. In the next stage, the pairs separate from their partners and migrate to opposite sides of the cell, where each one begins replicating itself. Eventually the cell itself divides to form two cells. At some point during this process of chromosomes separating from their partners, a no. 14 chromosome either breaks and unites with a no. 21 chromosome, or it becomes attached to a no. 21 chromosome without breakage occurring. In either case, an abnormal chromosome is formed—a 14–21 combination —and this abnormal chromosome will become a part of

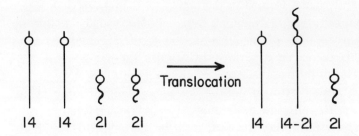

SCHEMATIC DIAGRAM OF A 14-21 TRANSLOCATION

the composition of the body cells in the person who inherits it. A person with this type of chromosomal abnormality would be a carrier of a translocation.

The translocation shown in the diagram is called a balanced translocation because all of the chromosome material appears to be present; thus all of the genes are present. The chromosomes are merely arranged differently, with the no. 14 and the no. 21 chromosome being joined. This abnormal chromosome will reproduce itself thereafter, but since none of the genes are lost, the individual with this chromosomal abnormality will be normal, both physically and mentally, but he will be a translocation carrier.

Either parent can be a carrier of a balanced translocation, but this defect has been more commonly reported in the female. The risk in this form of abnormality is seen when the ovum of a carrier is fertilized. In the process of fertilization (meiosis), it is possible for a cell containing the abnormal 14–21 chromosome plus the single, unpaired no. 21 (which was the partner of the 21 which united with the 14) to be fertilized by a sperm cell containing the normal complement of chromosomes, including a no. 21. The resulting fertilized ovum would contain the equivalent of an extra no. 21 chromosome. An individual with this cellular makeup would have D.S.

Statistically it has been found that, on the average, about 15 percent of the pregnancies of a female 14–21 carrier result in D.S. babies. The remainder of the pregnancies are about equally divided between normal children and other carriers of the translocation.

The importance of good genetic counseling becomes obvious in view of the high risk for the 14–21 carriers of producing defective offspring. Before the 1973 Supreme Court decision making abortion legal, translocation carriers were advised against having children of their own; adoption was the only safe avenue open to them if they wished to have children. Now, however, the outlook for translocation carriers has changed. With the development of amniocentesis, which made it possible to diagnose chromosomal abnormalities in utero, the translocation carrier is now advised to have children of her own if she wishes, but to have amniocentesis during the third month of each pregnancy to make sure the fetus is normal. If it is found that she is carrying a fetus with D.S., she would be advised to have an abortion. Of course, if she objected to abortion on moral grounds, she would be advised to adopt rather than have children of her own.

Translocation can also occur between the two no. 21 chromosomes or between the no. 21 and the no. 22 chromosomes in the same manner discussed in the 14–21 translocation. This is an end-to-end fusion of two small chromosomes, and it causes a more serious form of the disorder in that a much higher percentage of the children will have D.S.

The 21–21 translocation is relatively rare, but in cases where the two 21 chromosomes become united during meiosis the prognosis is poor. Recent research indicates that all of the living offspring will have D.S.

Although the translocation forms of D.S. are nearly always inherited from a carrier, there are rare cases when a mutation occurs and two normal parents produce a translocation D.S. offspring. Again, these findings emphasize the importance of cytogenetic study and genetic counseling for parents of D.S. children and their planning for the future.

For many years the medical profession was in a quandary as to what the role of the physician should be after the diagnosis of D.S. was made. Until very recently the doctor was usually unprepared to offer the family much help. Amniocentesis was yet to be developed. There were no classes in the public schools for trainable or educable mentally retarded children, and no sheltered workshops existed. The doctor was not even able to answer the questions of the parents as to whether the disorder was hereditary. Some doctors preferred to remain silent until the parents themselves realized something was wrong with the child; others felt it their duty to tell the parents immediately of the diagnosis, and to insist upon immediate placement of the infant in an institution for the retarded. Neither of these practices is considered to be correct at the present time. In confirmed cases, most pediatricians now feel that it is best to be completely honest and open with the parents. Those who are working in this field have found through experience that parents want to know the truth about their child's condition, and indeed they have the right to know the truth as soon as possible. The day has passed when the doctor made decisions for the parents regarding their children. In trying to shield parents from a difficult decision by making it for them, doctors were denying parents the right to decide for themselves what was right for their own child and for their own family. Moreover, it has been found that parents are better able to make adjustments and decisions if the doctor gives them the facts about their child. Today, the diagnosis is only the beginning of the physician's role. His first obligation is to inform the parents. If he does not have experience in this field, he should refer the parents to someone in this specialty. It is important that the initial conference be conducted by a pediatrician who is experienced in this field and can give the parents a simple, clear explanation of their child's condition as well as sympathetic general advice; above all, he must be willing to listen to the parents and answer their questions. At the outset it is usually difficult for parents to grasp the whole impact of the situation, so the first conference should not be too long or complicated, nor should the physician insist on any particular avenue of action. This initial period of shock and, perhaps, disbelief is not the time for them to make any decision at all about their child. Their questions should all be answered and they should have time to discuss the problem between themselves and with other concerned members of the family. It is usually necessary to schedule subsequent conferences, because the parents will have additional questions as they consider their problem and they may wish to bring other members of the family to some of these discussions. They should be told the advantages and disadvantages of various solutions, but it is especially important that they themselves make whatever decision is made after they have fully absorbed the impact of having a child who is "different." The decision that is right for one family will not necessarily be the right decision for another family because, obviously, every family is unique in many respects. Some families in which there is a significant religious influence may be able to work through the problem with the aid of their minister, priest or rabbi, and may not need a great deal of support from their physician. Parents who are emotionally immature may lean very heavily on the physician for moral support. Among people who are very family-oriented, the retarded child is nearly always kept at home, regardless of how severely handicapped he is; for example, throughout South America, there are no public residential institutions for the mentally retarded. On the other hand, a family with a different background may decide not to keep a severely affected child in the home. A few families may even decide on institutional care even for the moderately retarded child.

Most physicians consider that during infancy, home care, when possible, is preferable for D.S. babies. One important reason is that it is very difficult if not impossible for a physician to predict the degree of retardation at this early stage. Some infants thought to be severely retarded have developed well above all predictions when kept at home. D.S. babies are usually happy, playful and relatively easy to manage, and they seem to thrive and mature and develop to their fullest potential in a warm family atmosphere. It is generally agreed that even the best institutions cannot substitute for parental care. It has been found that those children who have had the advantage of home care during their early years are better able to care for themselves than children who have not had concerned parents teach them the basic self-help skills, such as feeding, dressing, toilet training and cleanliness. Many of them have also learned to perform useful chores about the house.

Professionals in the field of mental retardation, who have helped many families sort through their feelings to reach a decision about their D.S. child, have found that there is an advantage for the parents in keeping their child at home during the early years which many of them cannot foresee. Those who have decided on hasty placement of their child in out-of-home care usually suffer many doubts regarding their decision. Some parents may completely reject a child, but no matter how hard they try, they simply cannot "put an infant away and forget about it." They often have feelings of guilt for years. There is always the nagging question in their minds as to whether they did the right thing. If, after a few months or a year, the parents find that the presence of the D.S. child in the home causes a situation with which they cannot cope, they may decide on care outside the home. But this means that they have had time to get over the initial shock; they have had time to explore many avenues to help the child; they have taken time to rationally consider their actions, and to decide what, in the long run, is best for them, for their retarded child, and for the rest of their family. This period can also be very valuable to other children in the family in helping them develop healthy attitudes toward people who are different from themselves. Parents often find, to their surprise, that the presence of a retarded child in their family is a valuable experience, which has made them stronger and more understanding.

The following is an excerpt from a letter received from a parent of a retarded child. "I would like you to understand how much we all appreciate your help to us over these past years. Your optimism and intelligent guidance has been of enormous help to us not only in helping Gordon's development but in maintaining a competent family structure. I am sure that you recognize how tremendously upsetting a retarded child can be to an average middle-class Jewish family that places such a high premium on achievement. Gordon has learned a lot from us and over the years, we have learned an enormous amount from Gordon—what it means to truly love a child and accept his love without requiring anything more. It has truly been a lesson in humility."

If the parents have had the counsel and support of professionals in the field, they are much better able to make the proper decision for everyone involved—a decision they can live with and be comfortable. Such a considered decision can do much to free them from the guilt and uncertainty so often associated with early placement.

Parents always have added concerns about having a mentally retarded child in the home when they have other children in the family. It is natural that they should have questions about the effect on these other children of living with a retarded sibling. A study made of this problem suggests that it may not be too serious. It was shown that the attitudes of normal brothers and sisters toward the D.S. sibling did not reveal a detrimental effect on their happiness and welfare if the parents had good professional guidance and support. The study suggested that normal siblings not only closely reflected their own parents' attitudes toward the affected child, but they often considered him as a special problem and had no qualms in acknowledging this among their friends.

Another matter of special concern to most parents is the manner in which they should tell their other children about the fact that the new baby is "different." Parents who have been through this experience have found that a simple, truthful explanation is the most sensible way of avoiding further difficulties. The parents should impart not a feeling of shame, but merely the fact that Johnny is "slower," that he is just as much a part of the family as anyone else. This not only helps the other children develop a healthy attitude toward the retarded child, but also makes for their added personal security. The child who realizes that his parents feel love and concern for his mentally retarded sibling because he is a part of the family instinctively knows that his parents will continue to feel love and concern for him even though he may sometimes not come up to their expectations. Such an example set by parents not only gives the normal children a better understanding of the family situation, but it helps them to be frank and unashamed when they explain to their friends that their new brother or sister is "different."

Some parents may decide that care outside their home is the best solution for their family, and in some cases this is the best solution. For example, one third of D.S. children also have congenital heart disease, and some of these children need nursing care which is not possible at home. There may be other medical problems which make it difficult to keep the child at home. Parents may also decide on out-of-home placement when their marriage is unstable. The presence of a D.S. child in the home puts an added strain on any marriage, and in families where there is marital discord or where the partners are separated or divorced, out-of-home care is usually the best solution. In some cases, the mother is not physically well, and she may not be able to provide the kind of special care a D.S. child requires, and sometimes both parents are so disturbed that they are unable to properly care for a D.S. child at home. In some cases, when there are many other young, normal children in the family, the mother is simply unable to provide the care necessary for her retarded child and at the same time give adequate attention to her other children. There is no denying that the presence of a D.S. child in a home causes some physical, psychological and financial stress on the family at one time or another. For any of several good reasons, parents may consider placement of their child outside of their own home.

It should be made clear to the parents that whatever decision is made is not irrevocable. No couple should try to keep a D.S. child in their home if his presence is destroying the family. Their physician can arrange for out-of-home placement at any time. Conversely, there is no reason why parents who have decided on early placement of their child in an institution cannot reconsider and bring the child home. Professional counseling can help a family make these adjustments as easily as possible.

Parents who do decide on home care for their D.S. child sometimes feel at a loss as to how to help him. Since the condition is a chromosomal disorder, nothing can be done to correct the underlying defect, but there are many things parents can do to help their child develop to his fullest potential.

In many places, a new technique called infant stimulation is now being tried on D.S. children during early infancy. From first reports, it would appear that this technique does help retarded children become more alert. In 1973, several researchers reported on its beneficial effects on D.S. children at the first conference on Down's syndrome which was sponsored by the National Institutes of Health and the National Association for Retarded Citizens.

In such a program, the baby is given special sensory stimulation, on a daily basis. Brightly colored articles are placed over and around the child's crib, and special care is taken to place him in a position so he can see all the special equipment. Brightly colored articles are moved across the infant's field of vision so that he can follow them with his eyes. He is exposed to sounds of varying intensities. He is talked to and sung to. If the child makes sounds, these sounds are repeated back to him. Because an infant's natural tendency is to explore any sticky substance on his lips with his tongue, a small dab of peanut butter is put on his lips to encourage him to exercise his mouth and tongue. The baby is given objects of various textures to feel, such as velvet, sandpaper and metal. He is also placed in different positions and is moved frequently and exercised. Although such programs are still very new, results of studies have indicated that the infants do show marked improvement after such a program has been carried out.

It is important, however, for the parents to be actively involved in the infant stimulation activities. One reason D.S. children progress more slowly is that they are usually less active and less responsive than other children, so they need someone to take the initiative by providing extra stimulation to make them interested in their surroundings. They are often content to lie in their cribs or sit in their playpens for long periods without fussing. Mistaking this slowness and lack of alertness for contentedness, parents often report that they are very good babies. A busy mother is likely to leave the quiet, unresponsive child alone in his crib, and with D.S. children, this is the worst thing she can do. Parents who observe how this program is conducted should continue it by themselves. This is important, since the baby usually quickly regresses if the program is discontinued. Parents interested in learning about the technique should contact their local Association for Retarded Citizens or special clinics serving handicapped children.

Parents who are seeking ways of helping their D.S. children should be wary of the many people who profess to have special treatments and cures for D.S. It is important for parents to check with their doctor or local Association for Retarded Citizens before embarking on any such program, as many of these treatments are of no proven medical value and some are even harmful. Most of them are also expensive. Although medical science is discovering preventive measures and treatments for some forms of brain damage, unfortunately it still has not found a proven cure for D.S. No special medication or vitamin or exercise will remove the extra chromosome. Because doctors are busy with other patients and cannot hope to cure D.S. children, they may, in some cases, appear uninterested and the parents may be tempted to take their child to a practitioner who claims his special formula will achieve fabulous results. Occasionally children do show some temporary improvement while taking a special medication or treatment, but this improvement is probably due to the extra attention the child is receiving rather than the treatment itself. The parents are enthusiastic and expect the treatment to work; they give the child the special medication or vitamin or exercise; they may take him on frequent trips to the doctor. The child senses the enthusiasm and extra activity on his behalf, and he does sometimes become more alert. Unfortunately, the parents usually pay large sums of money for the treatment, when they could probably achieve the same results by simply enriching the child's everyday environment. (See the chapter on Unproven Treatments for more specific information.) The importance of spending time with the child cannot be overestimated—talking to him, playing with him, and taking him places such as the zoo, the beach and the park.

The best treatment discovered thus far for D.S. children is the combination of good medical care, correction of any physical abnormalities (such as correctable eye problems), good nutrition and providing a warm family atmosphere and appropriate educational programs so that they can grow and develop to their fullest potential with a feeling of being loved and wanted and needed.

The following story of Betty illustrates how one family dealt with some of the many problems posed by the birth of a child with D.S.

Betty M. was first seen at Childrens Hospital in Los Angeles at the age of seven months. She was referred for evaluation of a heart defect, which she had had from birth. At that time the M.'s were told that Betty was a Mongoloid (the term then in use for Down's syndrome), in addition to having a minor heart murmur. Their family doctor had referred the M.'s to the hospital because he had not known how to tell them about the diagnosis. Betty was their first child. She was attractive and sociable, and the M.'s had not realized that she was late in developing.

Betty was found to be a well-nourished, well-cared for, attractive infant, but she had poor head control and could not roll over. Her heart involvement was minor (many D.S. individuals have associated heart defects). There was no family history of mental retardation. The history revealed that the pregnancy had been full term, but labor had been difficult, lasting thirty-six hours. It had been a dry birth, and forceps had been used in the delivery. Mrs. M. also reported that when she was six weeks pregnant, she had had an emergency appendectomy. She had been given a spinal anesthetic, which had not taken effect before the surgery was started. Mrs. M. had gone into shock and was given stimulants as well as ether so that the surgery could be completed. The M.'s have subsequently felt that perhaps Betty suffered added brain damage during the pregnancy and birth, even though they know that these events did not cause the Down's syndrome.

When Betty was three years old, Mrs. M. gave birth to a normal, healthy boy. Betty continued to live at home, and developed normally, but at a retarded rate. Her IQ was later determined to be 34, showing moderate retardation. She was toilet-trained, and her parents taught her to keep herself neat and clean. When she was six years old, the M.'s enrolled her in a private school for retarded children, which she attended for two years. In the meantime the M.'s had become active members of a group of local parents of retarded children. When Betty was eight years old, the parents group started its own school for retarded children, and Betty began attending it.

As Betty got older, the M.'s encountered family problems associated with her presence in their home. Although they loved Betty and gave her every advantage, they felt that she was upsetting her brother. They also found it very difficult to control her diet. Betty loved rich food, and despite their efforts to control her eating she continually filled up on bread and cookies or anything else she found in the kitchen. D.S. individuals often have weight problems, and Betty continued to gain.

When she was eleven years old, Betty was admitted to Childrens Hospital in obvious distress. She appeared anxious and nervous, and was breathing very rapidly. Examination revealed that her heart rate was very rapid, and her pulse weak. Her lung sounds indicated congestion associated with heart failure. She was 4 feet, 10 inches tall and weighed 208 pounds. She was diagnosed as being in heart failure due to a minor heart defect and gross overweight— her heart was unable to pump blood to such a large area. She was treated with digitalis to slow the heart rate and produce a stronger beat, and was put on a diet of 1,000 calories per day. She stayed in the hospital for ten days and responded well to treatment. Upon discharge, she went home, where she continued on the diet. She progressed well on the treatment at home and her parents weighed her once a week. If she had lost weight, they gave her a reward, usually a piece of dime-store jewelry; if she had not lost weight, she got no reward. After she had lost 75 pounds, her heart was functioning well.

When the tensions between Betty and her brother continued to mount at home, Betty's parents decided they had to place her in some other living facility. They put her name on a waiting list for a state hospital for the mentally retarded. At that time, the waiting list was long, and Betty was finally admitted at the age of thirteen to a hospital about thirty-five miles from her home. Her parents had prepared her well in advance for going to the institution.

She knew she was going to live at a special school where she would have many activities, and where she would meet many new friends. She knew that her parents would visit her often, and that she would visit her home on special occasions. She adjusted well to the institution, and her parents became very active in the hospital parents group. A side benefit of having Betty in the hospital was the fact that she did not have free access to the kitchen, and she continued to lose excess pounds.

Although the M.'s had always felt she liked living in the institution, when Betty was twenty-six years old she signed a writ of habeas corpus stating that she wished to leave the hospital. Since 1972, California has had a law stating that residents of state hospitals for the mentally retarded may sign writs if they wish to live elsewhere. The main reason for the enactment of this law was that there was a consensus, even among state hospital administrators, that there were people in the hospitals for the retarded who did not really need hospital care. Many moderately and mildly retarded persons, and even some individuals with normal intelligence who had been misdiagnosed, were confined in the hospitals. Many of them had expressed a desire to live elsewhere, but were unable to do so because they could not get their parents' consent.

The writ was provided for Betty by a representative of the Regional Center for the Mentally Retarded. In California the Regional Center is in charge of all admissions to and discharges from the state hospitals for the mentally retarded. Betty's parents felt that the hospital and Regional Center personnel had been hasty in expediting Betty's desire to sign a writ. They felt that she did not fully realize what this move would mean. Betty had told them privately that she hoped she could go to take care of her grandmother, and they had tried to explain to her that this would not be possible (her grandmother was in a precarious condition because of her age and she would have been unable to provide the proper supervision for Betty). The M.'s were fearful that in less secure surroundings Betty might be taken advantage of or get into trouble, but they realized that the judge would probably grant her writ, so they decided to cooperate in helping with the move if a good facility could be located for her. Later Mr. M. expressed his mixed feelings. He had naturally been concerned about Betty's well-being, but he also felt that perhaps it was not right for a retarded adult to be kept in a facility against her will. Betty's writ was granted, and her parents worked with the Regional Center personnel to locate a good facility for her.

Within three weeks she was placed in a board-and-care home, where she is still living, in a community about ten miles from her parents' home. The residence was at one time a convalescent hospital. It has the capacity for ninety people, and there are supervisory personnel to care for the residents. It is affiliated with a sheltered workshop run by Goodwill Industries.

Betty adjusted very well to the change. She enjoys the added freedom. She shares her room with one other young retarded woman. She is pleased that she can have a job in the workshop and receive a salary for her work. She especially likes having a room with a dresser and closet of her own where she can keep her things. She can see her parents often, and they appreciate this also. Betty did miss her boyfriend from the institution at first (she said they had been going together for eight years), but after Betty left the hospital, her boyfriend also signed a writ and asked to go to the same facility where Betty lives. Although his parents opposed the move, his writ was granted, and he is now living at the same home as Betty does and working where Betty works.

The residents of the facility are free to come and go as they wish. Goodwill Industries sends a bus each day to transport them to work, and they are paid a small salary, which they can spend as they wish. The Regional Center has an agreement with Goodwill Industries by which the center subsidizes the employment of its clients who can appropriately participate in their workshop. The center has similar agreements with many other workshops throughout its area. In other words, if a retarded person under the jurisdiction of the Regional Center is able to properly perform the duties required in a particular workshop, the center will reimburse the workshop for the cost of that person's employment. In addition, the board-and-care residents are registered with the state for Aid to the Totally Disabled (ATD), which pays for their care at the facility. The work at the sheltered workshop varies, depending upon what contracts it gets. For example, the work may involve sorting or wrapping packages for mailing. Betty earns about $2.50 per week. Her supervisors report that she could earn more if she did not spend so much of her time socializing. Every Friday night, Betty and her boyfriend go out to dinner.

The M.'s still have some misgivings about the change. They feel the hospital and Regional Center personnel are overzealous in assisting residents in securing and signing writs. In addition, they feel there should be some sort of transition facility such as halfway houses between the sheltered environment of the state facility and the freer environment of community residential care. Mr. M. is a member of the area board of the Regional Center, and he worries that with so many retarded people coming out of the state hospitals, and with the amount of paper work and red tape involved in applying for ATD, unless each of them has a family or guardian to look out for him, some of them will become lost in the community and be taken advantage of.

The M.'s also feel that zoning should be revised to permit board-and-care facilities in better neighborhoods. They report that many things are stolen from the residents' rooms because the facility is in a lower-class neighborhood and the doors are always unlocked to allow the residents to come and go. They have also noticed that Betty has started gaining weight again because she is able to go to the store for candy and ice cream whenever she wishes. In addition, Betty has recently expressed an interest in sex and they are concerned that she may have sexual relations with her boy-friend now that they are in a less restrictive facility. They realize her sexual desires are natural and normal, but they also realize she would not be able to properly care for a baby. They plan to start her on the "pill" as a preventive measure.

Betty is fortunate to be living in California, as it is the only state at the present time which allows residents of state facilities for the retarded to sign writs. In the other states there is absolutely no way for a person to get out of a state facility for the retarded unless he has his parents' consent. The authors have seen individuals with normal intelligence in facilities for the retarded in other states who are begging to be released, but nothing can be done for them because their parents refuse to sign releases. In some cases, their parents are no longer living, and there is no hope that they will ever be released unless other states follow the lead of California in making the writs available to them. They will probably do so as they begin to see the benefits of such releases.

Another force which will be influential in changing the time-honored practice of locking retarded citizens away in institutions is the interest being shown by some members of the legal profession in the problems of guaranteeing legal and civil rights to the mentally retarded and the mentally ill. A new organization has been formed in Washington, D.C., called the Center for Law and Social Policy, and it is composed of lawyers who are interested in these very problems.

As more and more people leave the institutions for the mentally retarded, it is clear that there will be a need for many more sheltered workshops. Goodwill Industries already has these workshops across the nation, and other such facilities have been started by parents groups as well as by other agencies. It seems obvious that the mentally retarded should lead as normal lives as possible, and for many of them, an institution with a high fence and a locked gate is not necessary. Although the system being used in California is far from perfect, it is a step in the right direction and a beginning of normalization for the mentally retarded.

IX
Phenylketonuria, a Treatable Disease

Phenylketonuria (PKU) is a hereditary disease which affects one in every 10,000 to 15,000 infants born. Of interest is the fact that the daughter of the author Pearl Buck was found to be suffering from PKU. In 1950 Mrs. Buck wrote sensitively in her book *The Child Who Never Grew* about her struggle to accept the fact that her only child was mentally retarded. At the time she wrote the book she did not know the specific diagnosis, but this is not as vital as the good counsel she offers to all parents of retarded children.

PKU almost invariably causes moderate to severe mental retardation if left untreated, but during the 1950's and 1960's, in a series of dramatic breakthroughs, a diagnostic test and a dietary treatment were developed so that the disease could be controlled and mental retardation prevented.

The disease was first described in 1934 by Dr. Asbjorn Folling. He discovered that certain retarded children had a high content of phenylpyruvic acid in their urine, and that this could be detected in the laboratory when a sample of urine was acidified by the addition of hydrochloric acid. If there was an excess of phenylpyruvic acid in the urine, the mixture turned bright green when ferric chloride was added. Dr. Folling reported that children with PKU nearly always had very blond hair and blue eyes. They sometimes had a patchy type of eczema and a number of them had uncontrolled body movements and convulsions. Nearly all of them had a pungent, musty body odor, and many times they were hyperactive and irritable.

Dr. Folling's discovery spurred research on PKU, and soon thereafter Dr. George Jervis found that such patients had a hereditary enzymatic defect in which the liver was unable to properly break down phenylalanine (an essential amino acid present in all protein-containing food) into tyrosine and other substances which the body can use. When phenylalanine is ingested by a normal individual, it is converted to tyrosine by the action of the enzyme phenylalanine hydroxylase, but in the PKU victim, this enzyme is missing. Because the phenylalanine cannot be broken down, it builds up in the body of the victim and in some manner, as yet not understood, causes degeneration of the brain and resultant mental retardation. Phenylacetic acid, a by-product of phenylalanine, which is excreted in the sweat and urine of the victim, causes the typical musty odor.

Researchers theorized that if a diagnosis could be made before the disease had progressed to the point where brain damage had occurred, the use of a special diet low in phenylalanine would prevent the retardation. Subsequent research has confirmed this theory.

In 1953, Dr. Horst Bickel of Germany developed a special dietary therapy. As with diabetes, where the disease can be somewhat controlled but not cured by a diet low in sugar, PKU cannot be cured but can be controlled and mental retardation prevented by the use of a diet low in phenylalanine. A child who is already brain-damaged by PKU may profit by the diet because the associated undesirable symptoms, such as eczema, irritability, hyperactivity and convulsions, will disappear, making management easier. But once brain damage has occurred, complete recovery is unlikely.

Ten years after Dr. Bickel introduced the PKU dietary treatment, Dr. Willard Centerwall, himself the father of a mentally retarded child, developed the first diagnostic screening test for the disease. Dr. Centerwall discovered that the phenylpyruvic acid could be detected without first acidifying the urine as Dr. Folling had done. This eliminated the necessity of collecting a urine sample from the baby being tested, since the solution of ferric chloride could be applied directly to a wet diaper. If there was an excessive amount of phenylpyruvic acid in the urine, the spot of ferric chloride on the diaper turned green. This became known as the diaper test and it was the first step toward mass screening for PKU. Dr. Centerwall's discovery made it possible for doctors to do the test routinely in their offices without using a laboratory. This first diagnostic test was not accurate until the child was five or six weeks of age, but its development and Dr. Bickel's research sparked a flurry of activity in diagnosis, treatment and genetic counseling. Projects were initiated in which all of the inmates of institutions for the mentally retarded were tested. It was through this routine testing that Pearl Buck's daughter was diagnosed as having PKU. It was found that 1 percent of the individuals in the institutions suffered from PKU. In addition, it was found that while the incidence of PKU in the general population is about one in fifteen thousand, this ratio varies with different populations. For example, among the Irish and Scotch, the occurrence is as high as one in five thousand to six thousand, and among Blacks, Finns and Ashkenazi Jews, it is quite rare, perhaps as little as one in three hundred thousand.

These studies led to genetic counseling, for it was found that the birth of a PKU child occurs only when both parents carried a recessive gene for PKU. These carriers are completely normal, but among the offspring of such parents, one in four have PKU. Thus, with the identification of PKU victims, the parents could be counseled against having other children, or if another child was born it could be closely observed and tested for PKU with the knowledge that it was a high-risk infant. The siblings of PKU victims could also be tested, for two in four of the offspring of such parents were found to be carriers of the defective gene.

In 1962, Dr. Robert Guthrie, also the parent of a retarded child, developed a simple blood test in which an elevated blood phenylalanine level could be detected soon after birth. With the advent of this new and more accurate test, intense scientific and public interest resulted in the passage of legislation making it mandatory to test all infants for PKU before they left the hospital. California was one of the early states to pass such legislation. The test is inexpensive, but even so, there was considerable opposition to the legislation from the medical profession in California. Doctors feared that such legislation was a "step down the road" to socialized medicine, and the American Medical Association led the fight against its passage. Today, however, forty-three states require such testing, and screening programs have become commonplace throughout the world.

Continued research has revealed that more than one substance is required for the conversion of phenylalanine into tyrosine, and recently Dr. Sam Bessman has demonstrated that there are three isozymes (different forms of the enzyme phenylalanine hydroxylase) which have the ability to make the conversion. If one of these isozymes is missing, a small portion of the phenylalanine is not converted to tyrosine; if two of them are missing, a larger amount of phenylalanine remains unconverted; and if all three are missing none of it, of course, is converted. While all authorities do not agree with this theory, it does fit the pattern that is seen in the disease, and it certainly warrants further research and study, for varying degrees of severity are seen among the patients. Indeed, 2 to 4 percent of patients with the typical biochemical findings of PKU develop normal intelligence regardless of dietary therapy. With present knowledge of the disease, it is not possible for the physician to determine whether or not the patient is among these rare few, so the standard procedure is to put all infants with a confirmed diagnosis of PKU on the dietary treatment.

There are a number of factors which can cause an infant to have an elevated phenylalanine level, not all of which are PKU. Therefore the physician must determine whether the patient really suffers from PKU before instituting the diet. For this diagnostic procedure, the baby is hospitalized and serum (blood) phenylalanine and tyrosine levels are obtained. The baby is then observed on an evaporated milk formula (one part milk to two parts water with added carbohydrate) for two to three days to obtain additional biochemical data on phenylalanine and tyrosine in the blood. In the infant with classic PKU, the phenylalanine level in the blood remains elevated for several days after termination of the evaporated milk formula. If the laboratory data support the diagnosis of PKU, the infant is started on the low phenylalanine diet.

The basis for the PKU diet is a product called Lofenalac, a special milk food from which most of the phenylalanine has been removed, but which is otherwise nutritionally complete. It comes in a powder form and has the appearance of milk when mixed with water. For infants it is mixed in a dilution of one part Lofenalac to two parts water, with one or two ounces of milk added. This is used as formula, and as the child grows older it is used in the preparation of baked, frozen or cooked foods. Also, as the baby grows older, cereal, fruits and vegetables are added at the usual times. Fortunately, all of the strained baby fruits and most vegetables are low in phenylalanine. For the older child, cooked carrots, raw cucumbers, lettuce, radishes, summer squash, apples, canned peaches, pears, raw pineapple, raisins and rhubarb are all fairly low in phenylalanine. Some phenylalanine is essential, so the diet of the PKU child must be calculated very carefully, and phenylalanine levels in the blood are obtained each week during the first year of treatment. After the first year, the phenylalanine levels are monitored only twice a month.

The following is a sample meal pattern* for a six-month-old baby with PKU.

Breakfast	*Typical Meal*
6 oz. Lofenalac formula	6 oz. Lofenalac formula
1 fruit	7 tbsp. bananas and
1 cereal	tapioca
	2 tbsp. (dry) strained
	oatmeal

---

* Courtesy of Elizabeth Wenz, nutritionist with the Child Development Division, Childrens Hospital, Los Angeles, California.

Lunch

6 oz. Lofenalac formula
1 vegetable

6 oz. Lofenalac formula
2 tbsp. strained green
beans

Snack

1 fruit

3 oz. orange-apple-
banana juice

Dinner

6 oz. Lofenalac formula
1 fruit
1 bread

6 oz. Lofenalac formula
5 tbsp. strained peaches
3 tbsp. creamed strained
corn

Bedtime

6 oz. Lofenalac formula

6 oz. Lofenalac formula

In addition to these foods, there are certain "free foods," containing little or no phenylalanine, which may be used as desired. These include apple juice, certain candies, carbonated beverages, fruit ices, Kool-Aid, lemonade, Popsicles, Tang, Cool Whip, Rich's Topping, to mention a few.

About fifteen years have elapsed since reliable diagnosis and treatment of PKU became possible. The question of just how long the dietary therapy should be continued is one on which there is considerable disagreement. Some doctors feel it should be discontinued at three years. Others feel eight is the appropriate age because by this time the brain has reached a mature size. It may very likely be that each case should be considered individually, since there are individual variations in the severity of the disease.

The following case history concerns Jimmy, who had undiagnosed and untreated PKU.

Jimmy was four years old when he was first seen in the Regional Center for Mental Retardation in Los Angeles. He was hyperactive and fussy. He was not content to sit on his mother's lap or to play quietly with the toys in the waiting room. He threw the jigsaw puzzles on the floor and seemed uninterested in the picture books. He had no speech. He could walk, but was not toilet-trained and could not feed himself. He had been diagnosed as being severely retarded. The family came to the center seeking assistance in obtaining out-of-home care for him because his mother was expecting a new baby in six months.

Jimmy had a history of seizures, which were kept under control by phenobarbital. There were two normal older children in the family. The history revealed that Jimmy's birth had been normal. His mother felt that he had developed normally for the first few months. However, when he was not sitting up by eight months of age, she had become worried. He had started having seizures at ten months. He had been seen by several doctors, and a pneumoencephalogram* had been performed which showed that his brain was of normal size and shape.

---

* The pneumoencephalogram is a technique by which the brain can be X-rayed and it is an important diagnostic tool. Some profoundly retarded children are found to have very tiny brains, and in some cases no brains at all. Before the pneumoencephalogram was developed, it was very difficult to determine the exact dimensions of the brain in an X-ray because the brain was always surrounded by cerebrospinal fluid and it was difficult to differentiate between the fluid and the brain tissue in reading the X-ray. When a pneumoencephalogram is performed, the patient remains in a sitting position. A needle is inserted into the spinal canal and a measured amount of cerebrospinal fluid is withdrawn. When this fluid is withdrawn, the fluid surrounding the brain flows downward because of the force of gravity. Then a similar amount of air is injected into the spinal canal. Because the air is lighter than fluid, it rises and surrounds the brain. Thus, when the X-ray is taken, the brain is easily distinguishable.

The physical examination revealed that Jimmy was a well-developed, well-nourished retarded child with blond hair and blue eyes. His skin and hair had a distinct musty odor. Parents may think it strange to see a physician smell their child, but doctors in the field of mental retardation can nearly always detect the very distinctive musty odor of a patient with PKU. A serum phenylalanine level was obtained and recorded at 26 miligrams percent. This confirmed the diagnosis of PKU, since the average normal level is 1 to 3 miligrams percent. The electroencephalogram showed multifocal spiking discharges indicative of his seizure pattern and brain dysfunction.

The psychologist was unable to measure Jimmy's IQ because he was unable to do any of the tasks used to determine the intellectual level. He could not stack blocks or fit figures into form boards. He was unable to draw a circle or copy a figure drawn by the psychologist, and of course, could not converse.

Because Jimmy was so profoundly retarded, dietary therapy was not recommended. The diet is rather expensive and cannot cure a child whose brain has already been damaged. Since Jimmy did not have eczema, and his seizures were already under control, the special diet would not have accomplished much. Jimmy was admitted to a state hospital for the mentally retarded before his baby sister was born.

Jimmy's mother was alerted to the fact that PKU is a hereditary disease and that it would be of vital importance for her to have her new baby tested for this disorder before she left the hospital. She subsequently had a baby girl, who, like Jimmy, had PKU, but there is a happy ending to her story.

When Jimmy's baby sister was born, a serum phenylalanine level was obtained and reported at 4 miligrams percent. On the third day of life, the level was 32 miligrams percent, which was felt to be diagnostic of PKU. The special low phenylalanine diet was started, and at three months and again at one year of age, the baby was given a standardized trial of foods containing phenylalanine. These tests were closely supervised, and each time the baby was given these foods her serum phenylalanine level rose rapidly to over 30 miligrams percent, so she was continued on the special PKU diet.

She is now three years old and is doing all the things that any normal three-year-old does. Her last psychological testing determined that she had an IQ of 101. She goes to nursery school, but during snacktime, she eats a raw fruit or vegetable and orange juice, rather than the crackers and milk which the other children have. When she goes to birthday parties, she takes along her own refreshments of low phenylalanine cookies and sherbet which her mother prepares for her. The painstaking supervision of the diet of a child with PKU is time-consuming, but everyone agrees that it is worthwhile.

In studies where treated PKU children have been followed over a period of years, it has been found that they have a rather high incidence of visual-perceptual difficulties, which cause problems with academic subjects in school. These children often confuse such letters of the alphabet as *b*, *p* and *d*, and they may reverse numbers such as *6* and *9*. Such problems are also rather common to children with other metabolic disorders, and they may represent varying degrees of slight brain damage.

As the population of treated PKU patients grows into adulthood, these individuals will be marrying and taking a normal place in society, rather than becoming residents of institutions for the retarded as did their counterparts of an earlier generation. Of special importance to the female

PKU patients is the fact that unless they adhere strictly to the phenylalanine-restricted diet during pregnancy, they will give birth to mentally retarded offspring. The first such cases to come to light were those of PKU women who had not been treated and who were themselves mentally retarded. In 1963, Dr. Charlton Mabry reported on seven children born to three PKU mothers. All seven of the offspring were mentally retarded, although they did not have PKU. There is one documented case of an untreated PKU woman with normal intelligence who gave birth to four mentally retarded offspring. This discovery that maternal PKU itself increases the risk of mental retardation in offspring has complicated the care of PKU girls in that it is one more social problem with which these girls must contend.

The question which now must be dealt with is whether or not a female PKU patient should bear children. Obviously, retarded women should not bear children, since it has been demonstrated that children of mentally retarded mothers do not develop to their full potential and become retarded themselves because of the inability of the mothers to provide a secure and stimulating environment. The patient with normal intelligence should not be denied the opportunity of having a family. Unfortunately, it has proven very difficult for women to observe the phenylalanine-restricted diet during pregnancy because it usually causes extreme nausea. Most doctors now feel that these patients should not have children of their own, and should adopt children if they wish to raise a family. With skilled counseling, sterilization has been an acceptable solution for some. In the event that a PKU patient becomes pregnant, a therapeutic abortion is usually recommended. If this is unacceptable, she is put on the diet for the duration of the pregnancy.

In conclusion, while we have focused on PKU, there are several other diseases which can be treated in a similar manner, and undoubtedly as research continues, other treatable diseases will be added to the family of metabolic disorders which cause mental retardation. Galactosemia, hyperglycinemia, maple syrup urine disease, methylmalonic-aciduria, homocystinuria and histidinemia are all metabolic diseases that cause mental retardation. Screening is feasible for these and other diseases, and treatment is quite effective in preventing mental retardation. Some ten to twenty treatable diseases can be detected in urine tests, and another ten in blood tests. A few states have already initiated mass screening programs to enable them to diagnose all treatable metabolic diseases early in infancy. Massachusetts has the best program: all babies born there are given both blood and urine tests for a whole range of metabolic diseases. New York and Oregon have blood tests on all infants born; some other states are attempting to institute similar programs. If widespread screening programs for these diseases were introduced in this country, another step in the eradication of mental retardation would be accomplished. Each state should initiate such programs, but this will only happen if there is concerted citizen action.

X

A Team Approach to an All-Encompassing Problem

In dealing with the problem of mental retardation, physicians and parents alike have been frustrated and dissatisfied with the traditional "one man" approach which is usually employed by the medical profession. The physician is accustomed to diagnosing a disorder using a physical examination and certain laboratory tests and employing appropriate treatment to cure or alleviate the illness. Many times, when dealing with the problem of mental retardation, he finds that the customary examination and tests reveal nothing that would lead to a diagnosis. It has been estimated that in three quarters of the cases of retardation no actual cause is found. In addition, most physicians do not have the training to do the developmental tests to determine the degree of retardation. These are the tests used by pediatricians and psychologists to estimate the developmental age at which an infant is functioning. Although they are not predictive of IQ, they can indicate a pattern of delayed development, and they often forecast mental retardation.

Of course, in most cases, it is not possible for a physician to prescribe a treatment that will cure the disorder. In many cases the physician is simply overwhelmed by the magnitude of the problem presented by the mentally retarded patient, and, moreover, he is usually busy with more treatable disorders, so that he feels he does not have the time to work with the mentally retarded. Parents soon sense these limitations and become dissatisfied. They have many questions they want answered—and rightfully so: Why did this happen to my child? Is it hereditary? If I have other children, will they be like this? How long will my child live? Is there a treatment for him?

They may shop around, going from one specialist to another, searching for answers. They may become embittered at the whole medical profession, or they may fall prey to unscrupulous people who promise dramatic results from special therapies which are costly but useless.

Since the problem of mental retardation is such an all-encompassing one involving diagnosis, evaluation, continuing care and treatment, and family counseling, most centers for such disorders employ a multidisciplinary approach, such as that used at the Child Development Division at the Childrens Hospital of Los Angeles. To understand the way the multidisciplinary approach works, let us follow a typical case referred to the center.

A phone call is received at the clinic from a Mrs. Jones regarding her son, Johnnie. Her family doctor feels Johnnie may be mentally retarded. About a third of the referrals to the clinic come from physicians. The others come from other professionals such as public health nurses and school authorities, and some come from other parents of retarded children. Johnnie is three and a half years old and has not begun to talk. Mrs. Jones furnishes the name and address of her family physician so that the clinic may obtain Johnnie's medical records from him. Mrs. Jones is told that she will be contacted when the clinic has received all the data on Johnnie. The clinic always requests records from everyone who has worked with a child before starting its evaluation. In this way, the multidisciplinary team can have as complete a picture as possible of the patient and his background.

When all of the pertinent material on Johnnie has been received, it is reviewed by the clinic director, and an appointment is made for Johnnie and his parents to be seen in the office.

According to the case history, Johnnie has a sister three years older than he is. She is normal, and there has never been a family history of mental retardation. Johnnie was born prematurely at seven months' gestation following an uncomplicated pregnancy. He weighed only three pounds at birth, so he was kept in an incubator for the first two weeks. Subsequently he did well, so he was sent home from the hospital. He seemed to develop normally but a little slowly initially, which is normal for a premature baby. The family physician did not suspect that he might be mentally retarded until his speech failed to develop.

When Johnnie and his parents arrived for their appointment at the clinic, it was obvious that Mr. and Mrs. Jones were concerned as to the outcome of the examination. Johnnie appeared to be well cared for, but he seemed restless and nervous. The doctor began by taking a new medical history. Careful attention was given to the age of the mother at the time of Johnnie's birth, whether she had had a normal labor, whether there was Rh incompatibility or any prenatal illness, such as rubella. The doctor considered it significant that Johnnie had been born prematurely and had been very small. He questioned the mother regarding Johnnie's condition while he was an infant. Respiratory distress, feeding difficulties, jaundice, lethargy or listlessness are frequently early signs of cerebral dysfunction. Infants with mental retardation are often considered "very good babies." Johnnie's mother felt that he had developed normally, and said she had not become concerned until he was over two years of age and still had not begun to talk. Mrs. Jones revealed that Johnnie had been somewhat slow in attaining physical achievements, such as rolling over, sitting, standing and walking, but felt this was normal for a premature child. She stated that Johnnie had never had any convulsions, and that he had been physically healthy. She did say that she had been unable to toilet-train him, although her other child had been trained by the age of two and a half.

During the course of this interview, Johnnie wandered aimlessly and restlessly about the office. He communicated with his parents by the use of gestures and some infantile vocalizing. His parents seemed to understand what he wanted, although he used no recognizable words.

The next procedure was a physical examination of the child. He was weighed and measured, and the circumference of his head was also measured. Such measurements are important and should be done regularly to make sure a child is growing normally. Retardation in growth accompanies some types of mental retardation, and infants with repetitive infections can also be slow in development, although they may not necessarily be retarded mentally. The measurement of the head can be significant in that it may lead the physician to suspect microcephaly, hydrocephalus or craniosynostosis. The doctor did note that Johnnie had the narrow, elongated head which is typical of the premature baby. He did not attach much significance to this, however, as infants who are premature do not have the strength to turn their heads from side to side in the crib, and consequently the soft bones of the head become molded in a typical shape. This shape modifies somewhat as the child grows older.

The doctor carefully noted the condition of Johnnie's teeth. The condition of teeth can provide important clues to the state of development the child had reached when some stress to his system occurred which could have caused mental retardation. For example, prenatal anoxia can cause damage to the tooth enamel of the fetus. Changes in the enamel of the lower incisors may indicate a prenatal insult of sufficient magnitude to cause brain damage. Dysplasia (discoloration) of the enamel of all incisors is usually associated with birth damage, and generalized enamel dysplasia usually indicates postnatal injury from disease such as meningitis. Johnnie's teeth were normal, but the eye examination did reveal that he was somewhat far-sighted.

The doctor checked Johnnie for signs and symptoms of syndromes accompanied by mental retardation, but he found none. Johnnie did not have the low-set ears, the webbing of the neck, widely spaced nipples, simian creases (horizontal creases across the palms of the hands at the base of the fingers) and undescended testicles which usually indicate a chromosome disorder. He also did not have the odd face, heavy arched eyebrows meeting in the midline, limb abnormalities, deafness and severe mental retardation of the Cornelia de Lange syndrome. Like Down's syndrome, this disorder is characterized by a set of abnormalities which can be easily recognized, but it is very rare. The doctor also checked the size of his liver and spleen. These organs can be felt in the abdomen, and if they are enlarged they can be indications of other disorders which cause mental retardation. Johnnie's skin was examined for the scaly eczema which is a symptom of phenylketonuria and the dry, chapped skin which is associated with hypothyroidism. Johnnie's skin was normal.

Next, the doctor did a neurological examination. The purpose of this part of the physical examination is to determine the thinking ability of the patient and to check his coordination and various reflexes. Coordination and reflexes can give valuable clues to the physician regarding the seat of neurological and motor problems. Usually the doctor also makes through conversation and observations a gross estimation of how aware of his environment the patient is. Obviously, Johnnie was retarded in his thinking ability.

If Johnnie had been an infant, the doctor would have checked two reflexes which are important clues in diagnosing neurological damage. One is the Moro, or startle reflex. To test this, the infant's arms are pulled forward until his head is about a half inch above the examining table. Then suddenly the arms are released, leaving the baby momentarily without support. The baby reflexively extends his arms forward and outward, makes a similar motion with his legs, and begins to cry. This reflex is normally present up to three to four months of age, when it disappears. If it persists after four to five months, it is a symptom of brain damage. This test, however, is not used for babies over one year of age.

The other test that is always performed on infants is the tonic neck reflex. In the normal infant, if the head is turned right, the right arm and the right leg also extend, while the left arm and leg flex. The reflex is reversed if the child's head is turned to the left side. This reflex is also present in normal infants up until three or four months of age, and if it persists after four months, brain damage is suspected.

The doctor asked Johnnie to perform various tests of balance. He asked him to touch his finger to his nose with his eyes open and then with his eyes shut. Johnnie had a little trouble touching his nose when his eyes were shut. He asked Johnnie to stand on one foot and to walk on tip-toe and on his heels. Johnnie was unable to accomplish these tasks, indicating to the doctor that Johnnie might have some slight brain damage or delayed brain maturation.

Next, the doctor tested the deep tendon reflexes which give evidence of the condition of the nerves leading to the spinal cord. Johnnie had normal ankle, elbow and knee reflexes. The doctor also checked the clonus reflex. This was done by moving a tongue blade down the outer aspect of the sole of his foot from heel to toe. Johnnie's toes reflexively pointed downward. If his toes had pointed upward, Johnnie would have been exhibiting the Babinski Reflex, which is an indication of cerebral palsy.

The doctor also made sure that the cranial nerves were functioning. These are the nerves which carry messages directly to and from the brain. They have to do with the important senses of sight and hearing and they govern many of the movements of the face and neck such as blinking of the eyes, swallowing and sucking. The doctor held a vial of ammonia under Johnnie's nose to test his sense of smell. Johnnie reacted immediately. If he had not, the doctor would have suspected some damage to his first cranial nerve. He held a small pen light in front of his eyes and moved it from side to side and up and down to make sure Johnnie had proper eye movements. He examined Johnnie's mouth and throat to make sure it was not full of excess saliva, which would have indicated a poor swallowing reflex. He asked Johnnie to make chewing motions. Children with damage to the fifth nerve cannot close their mouths tightly. He made sure Johnnie could maneuver his tongue easily and that he could move his shoulders up and down. Johnnie did not have damage to any of the cranial nerves.

On the basis of the physical examination the doctor felt that Johnnie was a well-developed, well-nourished, physically active child who was somewhat uncoordinated. He referred Johnnie to an ophthalmologist for an eye examination to determine the extent of his far-sightedness, and to a hearing and speech expert for a hearing test. This is standard procedure in cases of delayed speech. The physician also ordered certain laboratory procedures, which are a standard part of the evaluation. In the laboratory the technicians performed a routine examination and phenyl-alanine determination on Johnnie's blood. He also had a tuberculin skin test and a urinalysis. A chromosome analy-sis was not ordered on Johnnie because he had none of the signs or symptoms of Down's syndrome or other chromo-some disorders.

Johnnie was then sent to the radiology department to have a skull X-ray. This revealed that the sutures in Johnnie's skull had closed normally. The X-ray would also have detected calcium deposits in the brain, early tumors and other disorders; the radiologist reported that the X-ray showed nothing abnormal.

The doctor also referred Johnnie to a neurologist for an EEG (electroencephalogram). There were other tests which the neurologist could have performed if Johnnie had showed signs of progressive neurologic changes, such as mental deterioration or loss of the ability to walk, but Johnnie had none of these symptoms. The purpose of the EEG was to provide a record of the electrical impulses of

Johnnie's brain. Johnnie had to be put to sleep for this procedure, not because it was painful but because the brain discharges during the process of going to sleep and waking up are especially significant in determining whether or not the patient has seizure discharges. So the Joneses made an appointment with the neurologist, and the EEG was performed the following week. The neurologist determined that while Johnnie did not have a normal EEG pattern, he did not exhibit seizure discharges. These discharges form an easily recognizable pattern which indicates to the physician that the patient either has seizures or is predisposed toward them, and may at some time have them. The doctor did not feel that the abnormal pattern was of great significance, as abnormal EEG patterns occur in 15 percent of the normal population, but they are more frequent among the retarded. The EEG finding was therefore considered to be only one sign, and not a diagnosis in itself.

The EEG is a useful tool to the medical profession in evaluating the condition of the brain. However, it is poorly understood by many people. This procedure, in which wires attached to the head lead to a machine which produces a wavy line, resembles something in a science fiction movie. The tiny electrical discharges produced within the brain are registered by the electrodes attached to the scalp, and in order to be recorded, these discharges must be greatly amplified. The line or brain wave which is produced on the graph paper is the record of the brain's activity.

Those of us who are accustomed to precise diagnostic procedures are often misled by the EEG. We are used to having an X-ray determine accurately whether or not a bone is broken, or a blood test determine whether or not a person is anemic, and it seems logical to assume that the EEG would accurately determine whether or not there is brain damage. However, the EEG does not have the accuracy of the X-ray or the blood test because there are many variables. First, machines vary in sensitivity. The other main difficulty is the interpretation of the EEG. Electroencephalographers can differ on interpretations: some of them find abnormalities in nearly all EEG's, while others find few. Another variable is the patient himself. The EEG of a patient may be affected by many things such as diet, amount of rest, illness, fatigue and drugs. These things can all cause an EEG to differ from hour to hour and from day to day. In addition, the accuracy of the EEG depends somewhat upon the age of the patient. The EEG's of children are more variable than those of adolescents and adults.

The most easily recognizable pattern of an EEG is a 9-to-12 cycle per second rhythm, which is called the alpha rhythm. This smooth, even wave is a normal tracing and is usually present when the patient's eyes are closed.

The purpose of the EEG is to determine whether the patient has a typical seizure pattern. The waves of this pattern are taller, sharper, less evenly spaced and more frequent than the waves of the alpha rhythm. A person sometimes exhibits such a pattern even though he does not have seizures. This could indicate a tendency toward seizures even though none have yet occurred. Sometimes an abnormal EEG pattern is exhibited which is not a typical seizure pattern. This could indicate some other type of brain damage such as a brain tumor or abscess, a subdural hematoma or a skull fracture.

Since seizures are caused by paroxysmal electrical discharges within the brain, and since different types of seizures produce their own distinct EEG patterns, the electroencephalographer looks for these typical tracings. A patient with grand mal seizures would usually exhibit a distinct EEG pattern, while a patient with petit mal seizures would exhibit a different pattern.

In a grand mal seizure, the patient loses consciousness and all of his muscles contract. He utters a typical sharp cry as the air is forced out of his lungs by the contraction of his diaphragm, and he stops breathing. During this initial phase of the seizure, the patient holds his arms tightly to his chest, and he turns purple from the lack of oxygen. When his breathing resumes, he alternately tenses and relaxes his muscles, and when the seizure is over, he falls into a deep sleep. Grand mal seizures usually last ten to fifteen minutes. Although seizures are frightening to witness, they are usually not harmful to the patient. It is important for the patient to be placed on his side during a seizure. If he is on his back while unconscious, he might choke on his tongue. There is one form of grand mal seizure called status epilepticus, in which the seizure does not stop spontaneously and the patient must be given an injection of an anti-convulsant drug. This type of seizure can be dangerous. If it is not treated, death can result. If a patient has a grand mal seizure while an EEG is being performed, the pattern shows a mass, diffused electrical discharge, much stronger than the usual brain waves.

Petit mal seizures, on the other hand, last only five to thirty seconds. The patient loses momentary contact with his surroundings, and his eyes may roll or blink. These seizures usually occur only about twice a week, but they can occur as often as every few minutes. The main problem with petit mal seizures in children is that they interfere with schoolwork, especially if they occur often. Occasionally a child has a learning problem because of the frequency of these seizures without his parents or teacher being aware of them. In such cases, an EEG can detect the problem and the child can be treated with a daily dose of an anti-convulsant drug.

Another pattern would be exhibited by the patient

suffering psychomotor seizures, in which he may grimace and chew. He may be confused and unaware of what happened. This type of seizure is sometimes preceded by an aura, or an awareness by the patient that a seizure is going to occur.

Another type of seizure is called hypsarrhythmia. It also has a characteristic EEG pattern. In hypsarrhythmia the patient extends his arms, and his body folds up in a lightninglike manner. It may last for only a few seconds, but it usually indicates serious brain damage or a metabolic disorder. Untreated PKU can cause this type of seizure.

Many famous people throughout history have suffered from seizures. An example is Napoleon, who, at the battle of Austerlitz, was confined to his tent for three days with a seizure and its aftereffects, after which he came out, surveyed the situation, ordered certain maneuvers, and won the battle.

Sometimes patients who have seizures exhibit normal EEG patterns. Therefore the person administering the EEG will use techniques to bring out the abnormal brain wave. Some of the abnormalities seen in psychomotor epilepsy can be brought out by sleep. The children tested at Childrens Hospital in Los Angeles are given chloral hydrate to produce a light sleep during the test. Certain other drugs can also be used to bring out the pattern. Hyperventilation (rapid, deep breathing) is another activating technique that is widely used to bring out an abnormal seizure pattern. It is important to bring out the abnormal pattern during the EEG if it is to be of any diagnostic value, because the type of abnormal pattern will confirm the fact that the patient does indeed suffer from a convulsive disorder. It will assist in establishing the exact type of seizure disorder, since each type has a typical EEG pattern. This is important because the different forms of seizures are treated with specific drugs. For example, a psychomotor seizure disorder would not respond to the same drugs as a grand mal disorder. If the patient does not suffer from a convulsive disorder, the activating techniques do not produce a seizure pattern in the EEG. Because the EEG's are more accurate when activators are used, they are routinely employed in most laboratories.

Occasionally, a patient may exhibit more than one type of seizure pattern. For example, he may have grand mal as well as petit mal seizure patterns. If a definite seizure pattern is discovered, the diagnostician will want to find the cause of the seizures, since they are sometimes symptoms of a disorder, rather than being disorders in themselves. For example, seizures are sometimes caused by a brain abscess, an infection within the brain similar to a boil. In such a case, treatment of the brain abscess is necessary in order to halt the occurrence of seizures. If, on the other hand, no cause can be found, they are considered to be idiopathic, and are treated by drugs. At present, there are many drugs that are used to control the various types of seizures.

In summary, the EEG is seen by the medical profession as merely one tool among many for the diagnosing of a disorder. To be effective, it must be administered and evaluated by a reliable expert, and it is never used as the sole method of evaluating seizures.

The doctor felt that Johnnie should be seen by a psychologist for an evaluation after he had been examined by the ophthalmologist to determine whether he could be helped by glasses, and by a hearing and speech expert to determine whether he was hard of hearing. Johnnie's score on a psychological examination could have been adversely affected by partial deafness or problems with vision.

The ophthalmologist tested Johnnie's vision and also

dilated his eyes so that they could be examined internally. He found that Johnnie could see well at a distance, but was unable to contract the eye lens for clear close vision, and he felt that Johnnie did indeed need glasses.

Johnnie's appointment with the hearing and speech expert went well, although he became somewhat restless and fidgety before the test ended. She established good rapport with him and he enjoyed putting on the earphones. She asked him to tap on a drum every time he heard a sound. She tested his hearing at all frequencies and volumes. Some children have a high-frequency loss and are unable to hear high-pitched sounds. Others have a more general loss. She found that Johnnie had excellent hearing. If she had found that he had a hearing loss, she would have referred him to an otologist (a doctor who specializes in diagnosis and treatment of problems of the ear) for an examination to determine the cause of the hearing loss. The otologist would have determined whether the hearing loss could be helped by the use of a hearing aid. Sometimes an operation to repair a broken eardrum or other damaged part of the inner ear can restore hearing.

A few weeks later Mrs. Jones called for an appointment with the psychologist. When his parents brought him in, Johnnie was wearing his new glasses. Mrs. Jones reported that he liked wearing the glasses and she had no trouble keeping them on him. This usually is the case when glasses really improve a child's vision. Johnnie was ready for the psychological examination. The psychologist asked the parents to be present while he administered the test, both to put Johnnie at ease and to explain the significance of the different parts of the test to them. The psychologist used the Gesell Developmental Test for Johnnie. There are a number of other tests he could have used, including the Stanford Binet, the Cattell Scale of Infant Development and the Vineland Social Maturity Scale. All of these determine the developmental quotient of a young child.

In the Gesell test, the child's progress is assessed in four areas of development: motor, adaptive, language and personal-social. The test takes about fifteen to twenty minutes to administer and score, and most children enjoy taking it. It is like a game, with the child getting the undivided attention of the psychologist. The child's motor development is assessed by his ability to handle blocks, and his adaptive (thinking) capacity by his ability to fit figures of varying shapes and sizes into a form board. For example, the child must figure out that a star-shaped figure will not fit into a square or circular form. This, of course, involves his visual perception as well as his thinking ability. He is also given a crayon and asked to imitate certain figures drawn by the psychologist. His personal-social development is determined by the way in which he interacts with the psychologist—whether he is fearful and shy or friendly and responsive. The child's conversation with the psychologist is one test of his language development. He is also asked to identify pictures, such as cars, birds, dogs and babies, in a magazine.

Johnnie related well to the psychologist, and began the test by stacking ten blocks. When asked to stack them again, however, he became distracted and would not continue. His father told him to go ahead with the game, but Johnnie looked restlessly about and tried to get down. The psychologist then handed him a crayon. He asked Johnnie to copy his drawing of a simple vertical scribble. Johnnie complied, holding the crayon with his thumb and forefinger, rather than with a more elementary, palmar grasp. He also imitated a horizontal scribble, but when asked to make a circle he merely scribbled again, and then seemed to grow restless and distracted. His father got rather upset with him and tried to help him make a circle, but this parental interference made him even more nervous. A simple jigsaw puzzle was then presented, but he squirmed uneasily and remained uninterested. He was somewhat more interested in the form board and succeeded in fitting the figures correctly after some trial and error, but when asked to repeat the performance, he soon lost interest, and became fidgety, trying to get down and leave. It was obvious that Johnnie's father, sensing that he was not doing well on the test, was becoming quite angry with him. Johnnie was unable to identify pictures in a magazine, and did not obey simple commands given by the psychologist. When asked to give the ball to his mother, he at first refused, and then threw it away. The psychologist found that Johnnie had a DQ (developmental quotient) of 70. In other words, he was functioning at 70 percent of normal for his chronological age.

The psychologist immediately discussed the results of the test with Johnnie's parents, explaining the significance of his findings on each portion of it. If he had had any doubts regarding any of his findings, he would have delayed discussing them with the parents until after he had talked with the physician and the two of them had determined their meaning. The psychologist recommended that Johnnie enter normal nursery school with two- to three-year-old children, and that a public health nurse visit Johnnie's home to offer assistance with toilet training and discipline. It was obvious during the administration of the test that there was a problem of discipline with Johnnie, and his mother had indicated that her failure to toilet-train Johnnie was causing friction at home.

About a week after the psychological evaluation, the clinic director made an appointment with the Joneses to discuss Johnnie's final diagnosis. By this time he had received the results of all the various tests, and felt that he could help the Joneses to better understand their son and plan for his future.

When Mr. and Mrs. Jones arrived, the doctor shared with them the results of all the tests, explaining the significance of each one. He told them that his diagnosis was one which might not be completely satisfactory to them because he could not tell them the cause of Johnnie's problem, but that it was a diagnosis occurring in 10 to 20 percent of the children evaluated at the clinic. The diagnosis was that Johnnie was a healthy, slightly hyperactive child with mild mental retardation of unknown cause related to prematurity and low birth weight.

Mr. Jones wanted to know whether Johnnie's condition was hereditary, and the doctor was able to assure him that it was not. Mrs. Jones asked about his future; the doctor told her that there were public school programs for the educable mentally retarded through high school, at which time Johnnie could probably find some simple type of employment and fit into the normal community, since he had no other handicaps, other than far-sightedness, which was corrected with glasses. He cautioned the Joneses against being overly permissive with Johnnie because they felt sorry for him, or because they felt he would simply never fit into normal society. He emphasized that the mildly retarded can fit in if they are properly trained and well-mannered. While he felt Johnnie's future was hard to predict, he thought the outlook for him was good. He told the Joneses not to hesitate to call him if any unforeseen problem arose.

The public health nurse began going to the Jones home once a week. She usually spent at least a half hour to an hour in the home, observing Johnnie and talking with his mother about his progress during the week. On the first visit, she gave Mrs. Jones a pamphlet on discipline and habit training for the mentally retarded. The pamphlet suggested firmness. It also stressed the importance of both parents discussing and agreeing upon certain standards of behavior for the child and then reinforcing each other so that he did not become confused. For example, if the Joneses decided Johnnie should not be allowed to scatter toys about the living room, this rule should be observed at all times and by both parents. Mrs. Jones should not show approval while her husband showed disapproval. It was suggested that discipline be applied at the time the child misbehaved, and not later, perhaps when Daddy came home. Various types of discipline were discussed, such as verbal expressions of disapproval, taking something away from the child, isolation and spanking. The nurse emphasized the importance of rewarding Johnnie for positive behavior.

As to his toilet training, Mrs. Jones was encouraged to take Johnnie to the bathroom every hour and a half in order to establish a schedule. She was told not to be concerned about the bed-wetting, as it is common in many children until the age of six to eight years. The nurse told Mrs. Jones not to expect instant improvement, but she felt there should be some improvement by the end of two weeks. However, at the end of the first month Mrs. Jones reported that there had been no improvement and she had been unable to get Johnnie into a nursery school because all the nursery schools required that a child be toilet-trained.

Mrs. Jones also confided to the nurse that she and her husband were having marital problems because of Johnnie. Mrs. Jones felt that her husband was very harsh with Johnnie, and Mr. Jones blamed her for not being able to handle the boy. Although they had not separated, the Joneses had decided to have no more children. The nurse felt that there might be less friction between them if they were able to talk with other parents with similar problems, and she referred them to a parents association for retarded children. They joined the group and found the social outlet a welcome one. They discovered that many parents had worse problems than they did. They also learned that the parents association sponsored a preschool program for retarded children in which toilet training was not a prerequisite. The Joneses decided to enter Johnnie in the school, although they were reluctant at first because they felt the other children were more retarded than he was. Those who worked with Johnnie felt that this was probably true, but that in terms of behavior, Johnnie was more of a problem than the others.

Johnnie seemed to enjoy going to school and his speech began to improve slowly. At school the children were all taken to the bathroom regularly as a group activity. Perhaps partially because of peer pressure, Johnnie quickly became toilet-trained. He remained in that nursery school program for three months, and then his parents moved him to a normal nursery school. Because of his delayed speech and short attention span, his parents kept him in the nursery school program for an extra year. He then entered regular kindergarten. He still seemed very immature, however, and the teacher recommended that he be kept in kindergarten for an extra year. Hoping that he had matured sufficiently, his parents entered him in a normal first grade the following year. However, after Johnnie had been in the class for two months, the teacher reported that he was still very distractible and just could not do the work. She suggested that he be placed in a class for the educable mentally retarded.

Mrs. Jones called the clinic at that time to see if some medication could be prescribed to "calm Johnnie down" so that he would not be such a problem in the classroom and could stay in the normal first grade. The pediatrician in charge prescribed a medication which usually helps somewhat hyperactive children. Johnnie's parents and teacher did notice some slight improvement after he was put on the medication, but he had fallen so far behind in the classroom work that his parents finally entered him in a class for educable retarded children. In the special education class, Johnnie's IQ was determined to be 66. He is still having trouble learning and is still restless and inattentive, but he is maturing slowly. His teacher feels that Johnnie will eventually be able to be self-supporting at some unskilled type of work, and he may even marry.

In presenting the story of Johnnie Jones, which is a true case history, we have attempted to show how the members of the multidisciplinary team function. The pediatrician takes the medical history and performs the physical examination; the laboratory technicians perform the various diagnostic lab tests; the neurologist determines whether there has been damage to the nervous system; the hearing and speech expert administers hearing tests and helps the child correct speech defects through the use of speech therapy; the radiologist does the X-rays which aid in diagnosis; the psychologist administers and scores the developmental and intelligence tests; and the public health nurse visits the home and offers assistance in the solution of various problems relating to the child and his family. Many times other professionals are included in the team.

The *social worker* is a very important member of the team, although he did not participate in the case of Johnnie Jones. Many families need more counseling than the physician has time to give, and this is where the social worker can be very helpful. After the diagnosis has been made, it is sometimes very difficult for a family to accept it, or the family may be unable to mobilize itself to follow through with a long-range plan. Sometimes one parent believes the child is hopelessly retarded and wishes to institutionalize him immediately, while the other parent refuses to acknowledge the fact that the child is mentally retarded at all. Some parents feel so keenly ashamed of having a retarded child that they can think of no solution other than immediate institutionalization. Others rationalize and think of reasons why the child has not developed normally; for instance, they may say, "He has a mental block against talking." Sometimes so much hostility develops between parents that their marriage is endangered. The mother may become so involved in her concern for the mentally retarded child that she has no time left to share with her husband, or in other cases both parents may become so obsessed with the care of the retarded child that they neglect their normal children. These problems usually fall within the realm of the social worker.

The social worker is a person who must be especially intuitive in sensing people's attitudes and feelings toward others, and is specially trained to help alleviate friction. Whereas most members of the multidisciplinary team are directly involved with the child, the role of the social worker involves standing back and taking an objective view of the child and his family as a unit. This role varies with different clinics. In some centers the social worker is the first person to interview a family upon referral for diagnosis, evaluation and counseling. In other settings, the social worker may become involved only if the family seems to be having so many problems that it needs special help. The social worker always takes a family history with special emphasis on the relationship of the patient with the other members of the family, and to the attitudes of the family members toward each other and toward the retarded member. In some cases the parents may see the social worker for several weeks on an ongoing basis for further counseling and suggestions for working through the problems posed by the presence of the retarded child in the family.

Often a child is referred to a mental retardation clinic when he is not actually mentally retarded but has a psychiatric problem, and sometimes the child is mentally retarded and emotionally disturbed as well. The experienced pediatrician can usually detect the child with psychiatric problems and refer him to a psychiatrist for treatment. Children who are mentally ill rather than retarded usually have no eye contact. In other words, they never look anyone in the eye. They look at the floor, out of a window, anywhere rather than directly at another person. They have great difficulty relating to people, preferring to involve themselves with objects instead; they may direct all their attention to the telephone on the desk or to a paperweight while ignoring questions directed to them. They are not affectionate children and do not demonstrate much fondness for their parents or playmates. At times they seem restless and agitated. They are often mute and have compulsive-obsessive habits, such as licking or smelling everything or walking on their toes.

In addition to taking a medical history and administering a physical examination, the pediatrician will usually order a test for PKU, since children with untreated PKU often behave in much the same manner as mentally ill children. He may also order an EEG and psychological test. If no evidence of mental retardation is found, or if the child appears to have psychiatric problems as well as mental retardation, the child will be referred to a psychiatrist. These children are usually treated by the use of play therapy, in which the psychiatrist observes them in various play situations to try to determine the basic cause of their problem. He will then counsel the parents as to how best to cope with such a child. He may also prescribe a medication to help the parents deal with the child's undesirable behavior. Some children are very destructive, gouging holes in the paper when they paint and purposely trying to break toys. The psychiatrist can immediately tell the parents that such a child is very aggressive and can advise them of the best techniques for dealing with him. Other children may adhere to a very strict routine in the play therapy room. They may play at first with the dolls and then go to the sandbox and finally to the paints. Upon the next visit, and the next and the next, they will follow the identical routine. Some children are so withdrawn and depressed that they may just sit in a corner and not play with anything in the room. It may take several visits before such children actually participate. Usually these children take little or no notice of the psychiatrist, so it is a hopeful sign when they begin to interact with him during the sessions.

The role of the *nutritionist* involves more than merely planning well-balanced meals, and it has become more important since the advent of screening for certain metabolic diseases. The PKU child must have well-balanced meals low in phenylalanine; the galactosemic child must have a well-balanced diet low in galactose. In the case of a retarded child who is grossly overweight or underweight, the nutritionist may be called in for consultation. If there is a child with a persistent feeding problem the nutritionist may make home visits to observe the child at mealtime and make appropriate suggestions to improve the situation. The nutritionist must be prepared to study the dietary needs of the individual patients and develop menus to fit their individual needs. Though not consulted in a majority of cases, this specialist is vitally important in others and is an indispensable member of the team.

The *physical therapist* usually becomes involved when a mentally retarded child has neuromuscular problems in addition to the mental retardation. Ten percent of mentally retarded children have cerebral palsy, which is a neuromuscular problem involving damage to the part of the brain which pertains to the child's ability to control his muscles. About three quarters of the children with cerebral palsy are also mentally retarded because the brain damage is usually not confined to the motor portion. There are a number of variations of this disorder. Some children are very floppy; it is difficult for them to begin physical movement or to maintain posture—in other words, they lack muscle tone. Others are spastic, and have too much muscle tone. Their muscles are nearly always stiff and tense, and it is difficult for them to change position or to maintain a relaxed posture. Still others are constantly in motion—moving their arms, hands and heads—although their muscle tone is poor. In some children the lower portion of the body is more severely affected, while in others the symptoms are more apparent in the upper portion. Some children have hemiplegia, in which only one side of the body is affected. In such cases, the child has normal control of his right side while the left side is paralyzed, or vice versa. And, in some children, all portions of the body are affected, including the muscles of the face.

The parents of these children are faced with many problems for which they are not prepared. To learn to handle a child whose every movement is difficult is a process that can be sorely trying to a parent. These children not only have abnormal coordination, but they have certain spontaneous, primitive reactions. For example, a very spastic child, when lying on his back, automatically pushes back with his head and shoulders, stiffens his hips, and often crosses his legs. Even when such a child is in a sitting position, any pressure against the back of his head will produce the same reaction of pushing back and stiffening of his whole body. Other children are unable to maintain their balance and must be constantly supported. Still others are unable to watch what they are doing with their hands; their heads automatically turn to the side when they try to feed or dress themselves.

The physical therapist is of tremendous help to such children, and is able to make many suggestions to their parents for dealing more easily with their problems. Since each cerebral palsy child is different in the type of involvement and severity of the disorder, the physical therapist must study the child and observe the manner in which the parents handle him. He can then develop a program to help the child achieve a better physical condition. Some children need more sensory stimulation; they need to know what it feels like to move. The physical therapist will therefore move their arms and legs in certain positions, which they find difficult to achieve by themselves. In this way the physical therapist can help them develop alternate movements so that they can function more easily. Other children are naturally sedentary and need a program of exercises. For a child who has difficulty keeping his balance, balancing exercises will be prescribed.

It is as important for the physical therapist to help the parents as it is to help the affected child. Most parents of cerebral palsy victims need help in learning to manage the child in daily living, because the afflicted child presents special problems in every area. He may be unable to keep his balance in a chair or he may be too stiff to sit down. He may have problems in feeding, such as having difficulty sucking; he may have a tongue-thrusting reaction which prevents food from being swallowed; he may have difficulty in chewing. It may be next to impossible to bathe such a child, and a never-ending struggle to dress him.

The physical therapist can provide many useful suggestions for coping with these problems. He can teach the parents how to make their home functional for their child. A special bath seat may make bath time enjoyable for a child who cannot sit with his legs straight out in front of him. Perhaps a simple suggestion, such as putting a baby on his side instead of his back while dressing him, may immeasurably simplify the dressing procedure if the child is spastic and stiffens automatically when placed on his back.

The parents will see the physical therapist first in the office, where he will interview them and examine and observe the child. Later he may come to the home on a number of occasions to observe the child in the home setting. And the child may be seen by the physical therapist several times a week.

In those cases where there is no mental retardation, the cerebral palsy usually improves as the child matures.

Mildly retarded children are often not detected and diagnosed until after they are enrolled in school and are unable to fit into the normal classroom. In such instances an *educational consultant* may be utilized. This consultant may suggest either an EMR (educable mentally retarded) class where simple academic subjects are taught or a TMR (trainable mentally retarded) class where the children do not learn to read and write but are taught to do simple household and outdoor tasks, such as bed making and gardening. These programs are both mandatory in the California public school system.

Occasionally, a child is placed in the wrong class or excluded from school for some reason, such as lack of toilet training or hyperactivity. In such cases the educational consultant can act as a liaison between the parents, the school authorities and the multidisciplinary team. As an educator himself, the educational consultant is much more effective in working with the schools than is a doctor or nurse or parent who tries to influence the school bureaucracy. The educational consultant is a person with teaching experience who is familiar with various programs offered by the public schools for the retarded and who can help in the correct placement of a retarded child in the proper program.

Occupational therapy is a specialty which started during World War I when our hospitals were filled with shell-shock victims and men who had lost the use of their limbs. Occupational therapy has elements of several other specialties: teaching, nursing and physical therapy. The occupational therapist has a good background in anatomy and physiology, and is also trained in the use of art and craft work which can be of therapeutic value to patients. He may teach alternative ways of functioning so that the patient, even though abnormal, may function more normally; for example, occupational therapists have recently taught quadriplegic patients to drive cars. The use of the occupational therapist in the care of the retarded is new, but it is becoming more widespread. They have much to offer in this field.

The *rehabilitation specialist* is usually associated with a sheltered workshop in which retarded people are employed. He may teach the employees how to perform various jobs, since workshops are not always involved in the same type of work. For example, a workshop may have a six-week contract to package products for mailing. Later, it may have a contract to sort the sweepings of aircraft plants and salvage usable nuts, bolts and small parts, which are then packaged for reuse. The employees must be trained for each operation to perform the work satisfactorily. Each step must be explicit and simple to ensure complete understanding by the retarded employees. It is the role of the rehabilitation specialist to organize these simple steps in an assembly-line type of operation so that, with group participation, fairly complicated tasks can be performed. Some typical sheltered-workshop projects include the making of rugs and candles and the construction of Christmas-tree stands. The rehabilitation specialist must be inventive and patient.

Other specialists become involved from time to time, just as they do with the normal population. Eye problems are not uncommon with the retarded, so the ophthalmologist is often consulted. The neurosurgeon may become involved in cases of craniosynostosis or chronic subdural hematoma, or in the placing of a ventriculocardiac shunt for hydrocephalus. The dentist cares for the teeth of retarded persons and the plastic surgeon corrects deformities of the face and hands which are common in some forms of mental retardation. For example, a cleft palate and harelip is a problem which is more common among the retarded than among the normal population; a child with such defects would be sent to a plastic surgeon for treatment.

Other nonmedical disciplines, such as recreation therapy, music, dance and physical education, all contribute to the care of retarded persons.

One of the main values of the multidisciplinary team is that through conferences the members can pool their knowledge about a given patient and arrive at a much more relevant course of action than can a physician alone. A conference of core team members is held on all patients referred to a clinic before the final counseling of the parents. This core team usually consists of the physician, nurse, psychologist and social worker, but it varies, depending on the case. Obviously, with a PKU patient, the nutritionist would be included, and with a child who is profoundly deaf, a hearing and speech expert would be part of the core team. In this way the parents have the benefit of the knowledge of each of these specialists in helping them make proper decisions in the daily routine as well as the long-range planning for their retarded child.

XI
Pseudo-Retardation

Pseudo-retardation refers to children who function at a retarded level but who in truth have normal intelligence. Several factors contribute to this seemingly incongruous diagnosis. The two major causes are environmental deprivation and emotional disorders. Other factors that can cause a child to appear to be mentally retarded are sensory defects, specific learning disabilities, neuromuscular difficulties and various chronic diseases. Except in the case of profound retardation, the true level of intellectual ability can only be accurately assessed by experienced professionals seeing a child over a period of time. No specific intelligence test is infallible, and it is only as good as the professional administering it. The profoundly retarded are usually easily diagnosed, since they are completely unresponsive. In addition, they usually have severe health problems, such as seizures and crippling disorders.

Not only are environmental deprivation and poverty responsible for a great deal of actual brain damage resulting in mental retardation, but they are also by far the major factors contributing to pseudo-retardation.

The environmentally deprived child who is pseudo-retarded will usually begin to function at a higher level when there is a change of environment; if left alone, it is almost impossible for him to achieve at his full potential. Over the years the damage will be just as complete and irreversible as if he had been born with 47 chromosomes or was brain-damaged by PKU. The tragic fact is that all environmental deprivation is preventable.

A landmark study was carried out at the University of Iowa by Harold M. Skeels in which the importance of environmental factors in relation to intelligence was demonstrated. In this long-term study, begun in the 1930's in cooperation with the Children's Welfare Research Station, State University of Iowa, and with the Children's Division, Iowa Board of Control of State Institutions, three groups of children were followed.

The first was a group of a hundred persons who had been adopted as children. Sixteen years after adoption, these individuals were interviewed. It was found that these persons were achieving at levels consistently higher than would have been predicted on the basis of the intellectual, educational, or socioeconomic level of their biological parents.

In the second study, a group of twenty-five "retarded" children were interviewed after a lapse of twenty-one years. Originally, as an experimental group, thirteen of the children who were in an institution for the mentally retarded were transferred at an early age to another institution which provided much more personal attention. Eleven of these children were later adopted. Twelve of the original twenty-five children who initially functioned at a higher level of intelligence than those in the experimental group remained in the relatively nonstimulating institution over a period of years. In an initial study, the experimental group showed a decided increase in rate of mental growth, and the others showed progressive mental retardation. In the follow-up, after twenty-one years, it was found that all thirteen of the children in the experimental group were self-supporting and none was a ward of any institution. The median grade completed in school was the twelfth, with four members completing one or more years of college. One boy got a B.A. degree. Their occupations ranged from professional and semiprofessional to semiskilled. One girl, whose initial IQ was thirty-five, graduated from high school, took one semester of college, married, and is the mother of two sons whose IQ's are 128 and 107. Eleven of the individuals were married and nine of these had children of their own. Of the twelve children in the contrast group, one died in adolescence following continual residence in a state institution for the mentally retarded. Three were still in institutions for the mentally retarded, and one was in an institution for the mentally ill. Among those not in institutions, only two had married and one had subsequently divorced. The median grade completed in school was the third.

In the third phase of the study, eighty-seven children of mentally retarded mothers were studied after a period of twenty-one years. These children had been separated from their natural mothers in early infancy, either voluntarily or by court order, and had been placed in adoptive homes before the age of two years. None of the natural mothers had achieved an IQ score of over 75. The follow-up indicated that the children were functioning well in normal society, and the second generation, or grandchildren of the mentally retarded mothers, scored average and above on intelligence tests.

Obviously, children cannot always be removed from their environment as these children were. But studies such as this point the way toward eliminating a substantial amount of retardation due to environmental deprivation. Projects such as Head Start are beginning to work in this direction, with the children being left in their home environments but being exposed to an enriched preschool experience. Head Start follow-up research in Los Angeles indicates that children who have taken part in this program continue to show higher school achievements than others. This finding is probably due to a number of factors. For one thing, the Head Start program has initiated a significant amount of parental interest and participation.

The following story of T.R. illustrates the serious effects of maternal deprivation on a baby.

T.R. is a two-year-old boy. His mother's pregnancy and his delivery were normal. The baby seemed normal in all ways at the time of birth. However, when T.R. went home from the hospital, his mother had no idea how to care for him because she was mentally retarded. Her parents lived in the East, so she had no one to advise her on the care of the baby. T.R. was left in his crib most of the time. His mother could not understand how to mix his formula correctly and could not afford a ready-made formula. She usually just mixed canned milk and water until it looked right to her. His bottles were never sterilized and she usually just rinsed them out before using them again. She did not realize that he should be started on cereal and other solid foods as he grew older, so he never got anything other than milk. She did not realize the importance of bathing the baby, and she seldom changed his bedding or his diapers, as she did not have a washing machine. Because of his constant crying, the neighbors became suspicious and called the authorities when he was three months old. The investigating officers found the baby lying in a filthy crib. The back of his head was slightly flattened because he had spent so much time lying on his back. He had not been bathed for two weeks and he had a severe diaper rash. He weighed only ten pounds.

T.R. was placed in a foster home, where he received good care. However, his foster mother reported that he was very irritable and cried constantly. Because she had other young children to care for, she had to give him up. He lived successively at three other foster homes, but each time he cried continuously and seemed to show no improvement. The foster parents all became completely distraught within a month or so of caring for the child. When he was eight months old, T.R. was offered for adoption.

He was adopted by a family which had three girls between the ages of eleven and fifteen. The parents wanted a boy, but the mother was unable to have other children of her own. T.R. was the only boy available for adoption, so the parents decided to give it a try. His adoptive mother was very calm and even-tempered and had been very determined to have a boy. However, even she was nearly ready to give up after T.R. had cried constantly for two months. He was still very thin and unresponsive. His mother described him as vegetative. He had poor eye contact, did not reach and grasp objects, did not sit up, crawl or stand, and did not vocalize. However, the older sisters were thrilled at the prospect of having a baby brother. They spent hours rocking him, playing with him and talking to him. All of this extra attention was probably one of the main factors in his improvement. He slowly began to change, making eye contact and starting to smile. Finally one day, he reached out and touched his mother. He began to vocalize and respond to the people around him. His motor development also improved. He finally started walking at twenty-one months and he began saying "Mama" and "Dada" at about the same age. At age two, he is walking well and saying several single words. He is affectionate and is functioning at about the fifteen-month level.

If T.R. had remained with his mother, he almost certainly would have become severely mentally retarded, if he had survived at all. In view of the fact that his natural mother was mentally retarded, he may also be somewhat retarded, but there is a good chance that his apparent retardation is due to the disastrous circumstances of his first few months and he will probably develop normally.

Robert Rosenthal and Lenore Jacobson reported in 1966 on their research at the Oak School in South San Francisco, that parental interest was nearly always a factor when children made good academic progress. Other factors noted by Rosenthal and Jacobson in their book, *Pygmalion in the Classroom*,* probably also account for some of the findings in the Head Start program follow-up. They found that the expectations of the teacher toward each individual pupil contributed significantly toward the academic progress of the pupil. In the Oak School experiment, begun in May 1964, a standard intelligence test was administered to all the children expected to return the following year. The test used was one with which the teachers were not familiar, and they were told it was the Harvard Test of Inflected Acquisition, and that results would predict which children

---

* Rosenthal and Jacobson, *Pygmalion in the Classroom* (Holt, Reinhart and Winston, Inc., 1969).

were destined to show a spurt of academic achievement in the coming year. The test was administered by the teachers, but was not graded by them. At the beginning of the next term, each teacher was given the grades that each child had received on the test. However, about 20 percent of the children were arbitrarily given high scores. These children were randomly selected, and their teachers were told that their high scores indicated that they should show a spurt in academic achievement during the coming year. In follow-up tests, which continued until May of 1966, it was found that those children whom the teachers expected to make learning spurts did indeed "bloom" academically at a higher rate than their classmates. The authors felt that the teachers communicated their expectations to those special pupils in many different subconscious ways. The results of this research combined with that of earlier research in this field do show proof that one person's expectation of another's behavior can come to serve as a self-fulfilling prophecy.

Just as a teacher's expectation that a child will make academic strides can be a positive factor in the child's achievements, a teacher's expectations for a deprived child can be a negative factor which helps to perpetuate a cycle of failure for the child. Teachers know that minority children and children from poverty areas do not do as well in school as middle-class children. Indeed, the effects of socioeconomic status on the scholastic achievement of schoolchildren are well documented in several studies, with those in the middle and upper brackets usually achieving above average and those in the lower brackets achieving below average. In studies by Patricia Sexton* in 1951, it was found that by the eighth-grade level, children from the

---

* Reported in Rosenthal and Jacobson, *Pygmalion in the Classroom.*

lowest-income families were two years behind the children of the highest-income families.

Teachers know that children from families belonging to a low socioeconomic level have language difficulties. Sometimes they come from non-English-speaking families, or if English is spoken in their homes, it is a limited form of the language. Such a child is immediately at a disadvantage when trying to understand the more grammatical and complex language of the middle class.

It is almost impossible for teachers not to be influenced by the actions and physical appearance of a child. The deprived child is likely to bring with him a distrust of others and a fear of new situations. He probably will not have been taught the behavior patterns necessary for school achievement. He will be noisy, undisciplined, and not ready to learn. His clothing may be dirty and in need of mending. All of this can influence the teacher. She feels the child will not do well; she therefore expects less from such a child. Just as a teacher will communicate her expectations for success in many subconscious ways, she will also communicate her expectations for failure. In 1963 M. Deutch* found that teachers in lower-class schools set lower standards than do teachers in middle-class schools. A. H. Passow* found that lower-class children are overevaluated on tests and grades, while higher-class children are underevaluated. In other words, teachers in schools in lower socioeconomic areas are tempted to set low standards for their pupils because they feel that the pupils will be unable to achieve higher standards. When the pupils do achieve at these lower standards, they receive good grades for their success. Therefore, a student in a ghetto school may get good grades but when he graduates into a school

---

* Reported in Rosenthal and Jacobson, *Pygmalion in the Classroom.*

or a situation where he must compete with children from middle- and upper-income areas he may find that his education has not prepared him to compete. And the child in a middle or upper socioeconomic area, who must struggle to keep up scholastically, may find that he is well able to compete with the best students from the economically deprived area.

As educators have come to recognize that poverty is a contributing factor toward scholastic failure, efforts have been made to enrich the education of children from poverty areas. Head Start has already been mentioned. In 1965, President Lyndon Johnson signed the Elementary and Secondary Education Act, Title I of which made money available for special programs for children of low-income areas. These programs include remedial reading, counseling, cultural experiences, parental involvement and health and welfare services.

Title I has been a step in the right direction in helping the environmentally deprived child, but administrators of public education programs must make these programs relevant to the children who need them. Unfortunately, a child is sometimes mistakenly diagnosed as being mentally handicapped, and thereafter, because of the computerized bureaucracy, he is labeled as such and put into classes for the mentally retarded. This can easily happen if a child starts on the wrong page of a computer-checked intelligence test, or if he is not well on the day of the test or if by accident he skips a page of the test. Any of these factors can lower his final grade to such an extent that he appears to the computer to be mentally retarded. An alert teacher must be aware that such things can happen and arrange for special testing and grade placement for such a child. In addition, through the use of restrictive entrance requirements, schools sometimes bar certain children. For example, administrators may require that all children be toilet-trained before they can attend any classes, or they may not accept children who are aggressive or have other behavior problems. Sometimes a particular school district may not have classes to serve children with certain problems, such as physical handicaps. These children must sit at home unless the parents know that it is mandatory that the schools provide an education for them, even if it means that transportation must be provided for them to attend appropriate classes in another district. The schools must cooperate in providing a good education for every child, regardless of his special needs.

There are a number of intelligence tests, such as the Stanford-Binet and the Wechsler Intelligence Scale for Children (WISC), which are standard measures of intellectual ability. In recent years, many psychologists and educators have been questioning the reliability of these tests in accurately assessing a child's intelligence. Many factors can influence the score a child makes: how the child is feeling that day, emotional and cultural factors, and language difficulty.

Studies have indicated that children who are raised by mentally retarded mothers also tend to become mentally retarded. The greater the degree of parental retardation, the less able they are to provide the support, warmth and stability needed for a child to mature normally. Since it is true that there is a relatively high proportion of mental retardation reported among minority families, some scientists in the past concluded that certain races were genetically inferior. Even now, at least two prominent scientists still espouse this theory. In the opinion of the authors, this is a simplistic theory which is simply not true.

Within the last twenty years, much study and research on testing has been done. At the present time, it is accepted by most professionals in the field of psychology that the majority of intelligence tests in use have been designed to conform with white, middle-class standards. For example, a child may be asked in an intelligence test whether bananas are yellow or black. To the child from an upper or middle socio-economic background, the answer, "Yellow," will be easy, but to the child from a lower socioeconomic background, the answer may be "Black"—perhaps the only bananas he has seen have been overripe black ones, or perhaps he is from a rural, disadvantaged area and has never seen bananas. As far as the intelligence test is concerned, his answer is wrong, but when his background is taken into consideration, his answer is perfectly understandable. Thus, under the present system, the culturally deprived child or the child from a different cultural environment is at a disadvantage, and consequently scores lower on the intelligence test. If, on the other hand, the tests were devised to conform to the cultural standards of certain minorities, the white middle-class child would be at a disadvantage and would achieve a lower score. For example, very few white middle-class children would be able to correctly answer questions about collard greens and chitlings.

Intelligence tests will become reliable in indicating the true abilities of all children only when racial prejudice and discrimination have been eliminated from society as a whole, and when the poverty and ill health associated with prejudice can also be eliminated.

Besides the fact that children from other than white middle-class backgrounds are at a disadvantage when taking a standard intelligence test, their lower scores are probably partially attributable to the degradation suffered by certain minority races.

The Black and the American Indian, especially, have been made to feel inferior by the ruling majority. Such domination and subjugation can so dehumanize the spirit of a people as to cause psychological damage which persists generation after generation. David Wechsler defines intelligence as "the aggregate or global capacity of an individual to act purposefully, to think rationally and to deal effectively with his environment." When this definition is applied to many of our minority citizens, one can see how disadvantaged they are in the environment of the white majority. Since our society is so divided, with people of different cultures isolated and insulated from each other, the minority citizens, while they may function very effectively in the limited environment of their immediate neighborhood, are unable to do so in the environment created by the white majority. It is this environment of the white majority in which they must compete and with which they must deal. The citizen whose native language is not English is obviously at a disadvantage, and there are those who, because of their race, have been denied many of their fundamental rights. These people have literally been prevented from acting purposefully or dealing effectively with the environment.

The suffering of the American Indian at the hands of the white man has truly been devastating. The Indian child of today bears the scars of the time when "the only good Indian was a dead Indian." In one study of Paiute Indian children in Bishop, California, conducted by Drs. Richard Koch and Karol Fishler, all of the Indian children during a period of four years were routinely examined for medical problems, growth patterns and intellectual ability. Of all the children studied, only one child was found to be truly mentally retarded. The others were all alert, bright-appearing children. However, the usual pattern of progress in school for Indian children in Bishop had been for them to pass easily through grade school, but to begin to fall behind and to drop out at the junior and senior high school level. By graduation time, 90 percent of them had usually dropped out. Since the children were not mentally retarded, this high rate of poor achievement was attributed to several environmental factors. The Indian families were still living on reservation land, and many were on welfare. Tuberculosis and alcoholism were serious problems in many families. Housing was poor and many of the children suffered from recurrent ear and respiratory infections related to poor food habits and inadequate heating in their homes. As part of the study, an enriched prekindergarten program was instituted for these children. They attended school each day in a bright, cheerful room equipped with attractive furniture, toys and books. They received a great deal of personal attention because there was a teacher and an aide for every twelve children; at lunchtime, they were given a hot meal. It was hoped this program would be a helpful factor, which would benefit them in the classroom as they grew older. Although the project ended prematurely because of the loss of a federal grant, and no final proof was obtained, it was felt that those Indian children who had participated in the program would be better able to compete with the white children in the higher grades in school. It appeared that the main reason for the history of poor Indian achievement in the Bishop schools was peer pressure and other social factors rather than any actual inability to compete academically with the white children. In other words, over the years the Indian children had entered school poorly fed and clothed, coming from substandard houses. As they grew older, they became increasingly aware of the discrepancy between their environment and the background of the white children, and eventually withdrew and stopped trying to compete. They probably got little encouragement from their parents to continue in school, and possibly they were criticized by fellow Indian students for conforming to white standards. The overriding factor seemed to be the inability of the Indians to successfully compete in a culture oriented toward the white middle class. This failure is undoubtedly related to the historical domination of the Indian by the white man and to the discrimination, much of which is subconscious, that exists even today in our society. The many movies about cowboys and Indians on television in which the Indians are usually the "bad guys," or at least, the stupid guys, certainly continue the denigration of Indian values and culture.

In the case of the Black American, the malignant institution of slavery so etched the concept of white superiority and white supremacy into every aspect of the nation's consciousness that these same distorted views still permeate our society. While this sickness of racism had produced subconscious fear and guilt among white people, it has been altogether shattering to the Black citizens, whose heritage is despair and self-depreciation.

Probably one of the biggest contributors to environmental deprivation is the cultural separation which exists today because of our housing patterns. In the South, this separation was, of course, ordained by law. In the North, it was adhered to almost as strictly as if it had been the law of the land. For years we have complacently ignored the fact that our minority citizens are consigned to the older, deteriorating parts of our cities where they live in overcrowded, unsanitary conditions. We have subscribed to generalizations which have no basis in fact. For example, it has often been said, "They [minorities] ruin property values. Whenever one moves into a neighborhood, others follow and the houses become shabby and neglected." This statement completely ignores the fact that minorities have never been allowed in a neighborhood until it has already started to decline. Then, as others have moved in, it is assumed that the decline is caused by the minorities, rather than that the decline is just a continuation of a trend which had already started. We have also heard it said, "They [Blacks, Chicanos] live as they do because they like it that way." In truth, no one likes living in a deteriorating slum neighborhood.

In the past, minorities have been discriminated against in every way regarding housing. Not only Blacks and Chicanos were discriminated against, but Orientals as well. The United States Immigration and Naturalization Act, passed in the 1920's, singled out certain nationalities which were ineligible for naturalization. These included Chinese, Japanese, Koreans, Indians and a number of other Oriental peoples. And in eleven Western states, the Alien Land Laws were enforced, which said that no person could own land who was not eligible for citizenship. Therefore the only people in these ethnic groups who could own real estate were those who were born in this country or individuals who became citizens by special acts of Congress. In 1943, Chinese people were granted the right to become naturalized citizens. The Alien Land Laws did not become null and void until 1952.

It was not until 1948 that the Supreme Court struck down the use of restrictive covenants in the sale of property. By 1950 the Federal Housing Administration (FHA) had modified its underwriting policies, which had been highly discriminatory, to comply with the Supreme Court ruling. In 1962 President John F. Kennedy signed Executive Order 11063 extending FHA financing to Blacks who wanted to buy homes outside of all Black areas.

In the past, banks routinely turned down loans to people of minority races, or offered them less attractive financing (high interest rates and short-term loans). Real estate agents refused to show them housing in other than Black neighborhoods, and landlords in white areas refused to rent to them. Most property deeds carried racial restrictions. It is little wonder that the ghetto exists as it does today. Tom Wicker was correct when he stated in his introduction to the Report of the National Advisory Commission on Civil Disorders, "What white Americans have never fully understood—but what the Negro can never forget—is that white society is deeply implicated in the ghetto. White institutions created it, white institutions maintain it, and white society condones it."

Even with the civil rights legislation of 1964 making it illegal to discriminate because of race, discrimination still goes on, sometimes overt, sometimes hidden. The Department of Housing and Urban Development, the Fair Employment Practices Commission and the Justice Department are all empowered to enforce the laws of equal opportunity in real estate renting, selling and lending, but these agencies are all so understaffed that they provide little more than token enforcement. Complaints must be handled on a first-come, first-served basis, which means people must wait. As one fair housing council director remarked, "Investigating discrimination in housing is like investigating a rotten tomato. It must be done when the complaint comes in, not two weeks hence, or it disappears." Even if an individual or firm is convicted for discriminatory practices, the law has very poor teeth and the penalties are minimal. Moreover, the government in recent years has demonstrated a reluctance to be more than remotely involved in this area.

Actually, the job of investigating complaints, attempting reconciliations with landlords who discriminate, and assisting those discriminated against in filing suits has fallen, in large part, to voluntary fair housing groups, which receive little or no governmental financing. Even though these fair housing groups face a continual struggle to raise funds, they do accomplish results. One such organization in Los Angeles, the Westside Fair Housing Council, operates with one paid employee and some two hundred volunteers. In all, there are ten such groups operating in Southern California under an umbrella organization called the Fair Housing Congress of Southern California.

Unfortunately the timid steps taken by the government and the hard work of voluntary fair housing organizations to bring about integration have failed to end segregation in our cities. This is tragic because segregation has contributed toward the environmental deprivation of the minorities and the poor, and these factors in turn have caused mental retardation.

The Supreme Court enunciated in *Brown v. the Board of Education*:

We come then to the question presented: Does segregation of children in public schools solely on the basis of race, even though the physical facilities and other "tangible" factors may be equal, deprive the children of the minority group of equal educational opportunities? We believe that it does.

. . . To separate them from others of similar age and qualifications solely because of their race generates a feeling of inferiority as to their status in the community that may affect their hearts and minds in a way unlikely ever to be undone . . .

Segregation of white and colored children in public schools has a detrimental effect upon the colored children. The impact is greater when it has the sanction of the law: for the policy of separating the races is usually interpreted as denoting the inferiority of the Negro group. A sense of inferiority affects the motivation of a child to learn. Segregation with the sanction of law, therefore, has a tendency to retard the educational and mental development of Negro children and to deprive them of some of the benefits they would receive in a racially integrated school system . . .

We conclude that in the field of public education, the doctrine of "separate but equal" has no place. Therefore, we hold that the plaintiffs and others similarly situated for whom the actions have been brought are, by reason of segregation complained of, deprived of the equal protection of the laws guaranteed by the Fourteenth Amendment.

Bussing has been used for years to maintain segregation in the schools; it is now being advocated as a means of achieving integration. True, bussing is one method by which the pattern of segregation can be altered until every man can live in the location of his choice. However, although integrated schools are certainly to be desired and bussing can help to achieve them, the minority child who is bussed out of his slum environment to school each morning and back again in the afternoon is not getting the complete change of environment needed to alleviate cultural deprivation. In the opinion of the authors, it is not the bus ride which is damaging to the child, as opponents of bussing try to point out—in fact, for children from a deprived, unhappy environment, a bus ride is probably preferable to extra time spent at home; it is the fact that the child does not ever really get away from the slum that produces the damage.

We agree with John Caughey's statement in *To Kill a Child's Spirit** that logic and testing indicate that integration would improve academic achievement, while common sense and the sociologists add a broader educational endorsement, saying that the integrated school would better prepare all young people, white and black, for life and usefulness in America's multiracial society. In this context it is

---

* John Caughey: *To Kill a Child's Spirit* (Itasca, Ill., F.E. Peacock Publishers, Inc., 1973).

encouraging to see that social change is occurring, though sometimes in ways that are shocking and ugly. While disturbing and threatening to the white establishment, the riots of the 1960's were a healthy sign: they led to the extensive investigations by the National Advisory Commission on Civil Disorders and the ultimate acknowledgment that ours is a racist society. True, the confrontations were bloody and lives were lost and property was damaged, but the American Black had gained sufficient pride and self-confidence to fight back rather than continue to suffer the inequality and indignity that had been his lot. The Mexican-Americans, too, have gained a new self-pride, and have challenged many of the practices which discriminated against them. And now, in the 1970's, the American Indian has a new self-awareness and has begun resorting to militancy.

In our view, the answer to the many problems of racial inequality lies in the field of housing. The problem of environmental deprivation will not be solved until there is adequate housing available in each community for families of all income levels, and when each person is able to live in the location of his choice. The availability of low-cost housing in all sections of our cities would help to achieve this goal; a person of low income would then be able to live in the locality where he is employed, even if it is a middle- or upper-income community. His children would attend the local school and perhaps escape the cycle of cultural deprivation that poverty and segregation have thus far ensured. It is simplistic to believe that merely changing housing patterns will completely solve the problem of cultural deprivation, but it will be a very large step in the right direction.

While this is a difficult period, with most of the white middle-class attitudes being challenged, and with such militancy on the part of some minority citizens that they are accused of racism in reverse, it is a time when minorities are gaining a healthy self-respect and cultural pride. It is a time of emotional growth and maturity for our society, and out of it should come a stronger nation—one in which children will not fail in school because of self-depreciation and self-hatred.

Emotional or psychiatric disorders can often cause a child to seem mentally retarded. Some children are very immature and hyperactive, and although they have normal and sometimes superior intelligence, their attention span is so short that they fall behind in their schoolwork. In addition, emotionally disturbed children are often given tranquilizers, which tend to dull their responses to the various items on intelligence tests. Children whose home situation is unhappy may find themselves so preoccupied with their home problems that they are unable to concentrate on their classwork. The schizophrenic child who is mute and withdrawn may have normal intelligence, but his emotional problem makes it impossible to properly administer an intelligence test, and, of course, the results of such a test will indicate mental retardation. For most children with emotional problems, standard intelligence tests are inappropriate in that they create situations of stress and these children already suffer from chronic anxiety. About 10 percent of the children referred to the Regional Center for Mental Retardation in Los Angeles are actually emotionally disturbed. Often it is difficult to tell whether a child is retarded or emotionally disturbed, and, of course, sometimes he is both retarded and emotionally disturbed. The experienced physician usually looks for certain clues. For example, the emotionally disturbed child often has parents who are also disturbed. He avoids eye contact, while the retarded child usually does not. The disturbed child is unaffectionate, while the retarded child is often very affectionate. And the emotionally disturbed child is often anxious and nervous, while the retarded child is usually relaxed.

Such children are usually referred to a psychiatrist, a psychiatric social worker or a clinical psychologist for treatment. They may also be referred to one of a number of community groups and church agencies which now offer counseling and treatment. These include such organizations as the Jewish Big Brothers, the Catholic Social Service Agencies and the local community mental health clinics.

Other children who may appear to be mentally retarded although they are normal in intelligence are those with sensory disorders. Obviously, children who do not see or hear normally cannot achieve academically at the same rate as others unless they have special help. Sometimes in such cases, the more intelligent the child is, the more difficult it is for the physician to correctly diagnose the disorder, for such a child will devise alternative ways of functioning to make up for his disability. The parents and the child's physician, while aware of unusual behavior patterns and slow development, may not realize the causal disorders. For example, a child with poor eyesight may appear normal in many respects, but he will be clumsy, falling over objects on the floor or running into things. He will not enjoy picture books as normal children do, and, of course, he will not learn to read. But he may enjoy listening to music and having stories read to him, as any other child would. In such cases, unless the parents are unusually observant, they may not realize that he has a basic problem of poor eyesight. This is especially true of far-sighted children.

Children who are hard of hearing can often mask their

disorders in such ways that a correct diagnosis is also difficult. Some very intelligent children who are hard of hearing even teach themselves to lip-read, making diagnosis doubly difficult. Occasionally, the child's teacher may be the first to suspect the correct diagnosis. Sometimes a clear-cut diagnosis cannot be made until the child has been seen by a physician several times over a period of several months or even years.

Sensory defects are usually congenital. They can be caused by a multitude of conditions, such as maternal illness or heredity. Often these handicaps occur together in a child. Some multiply-handicapped children are blind and deaf, while others are deaf and have seizures. Still others are blind and emotionally disturbed. These multiply-handicapped children are very apt to appear to be mentally retarded. Physicians and psychologists must be very careful in evaluating them.

The following story of Janet R., a multiply-handicapped child, illustrates the importance of home care for infants thought to be mentally retarded and of continuing testing and evaluation, for diagnoses can be wrong. It shows what can be accomplished when parents have the determination to challenge the opinions of professionals when they feel they are wrong, and the determination and patience to work with them when they feel they are right. Janet was diagnosed as being profoundly mentally retarded and her parents were even advised at one point to apply for her placement in a state hospital for the mentally retarded. Today, she is attending a junior high school for normal children, and is getting above average grades.

Janet R. was referred to Childrens Hospital at the age of three months because she exhibited many abnormal signs and symptoms. According to the family history, she had four normal older sisters. Her mother reported that her pregnancy had been full term, but that she had taken two tranquilizers when she was in the third month to try to control the severe nausea brought on by a persistent inner-ear infection which affected her sense of balance. Because of an adverse reaction to the medication, she did not take it again. When the infection cleared up, her balance became normal and her "seasickness" disappeared. However, she feels strongly that the use of the tranquilizers could have caused Janet's problem. Since that time, one of the drugs has been disapproved for use during pregnancy.

Mrs. R. felt from the beginning that the baby was different from her other babies, and by the time Janet was one month old she was sure something was wrong. The baby had trouble nursing. She was unresponsive and did not smile. Her parents were unable to comfort her except by holding her.

The physical examination revealed a well-developed but thin infant. She did not vocalize or roll over. She also had nystagmus, a condition in which the eyes quiver, and she had no head control. In addition, she had no Moro reflex. These signs led the physician to suspect brain damage. He felt she was mentally retarded, as well as exhibiting early signs of athetoid cerebral palsy, as she had some of the symptoms of this neuromuscular disorder. Cerebral palsy is characterized by writhing movements of the arms and legs, a tremor of the hands when reaching or working, poor balance and poor coordination.

At home, Mrs. R. began placing Janet on the floor and putting her toys in front of her to keep her contented. Even though Janet was unable to lift her head off the floor, she reached for the toys and enjoyed handling them. Mrs. R. also found that she enjoyed feeling materials of different textures, such as velvet and satin. When the baby was ten months old, Mrs. R. suddenly discovered that she was exhibiting a Moro reflex, and from that time on she felt that the baby began to develop better balance and head control. However, when she was seen at one year of age at Childrens Hospital, she still did not have good head control, and according to the Gesell Developmental Scale, she had a DQ (developmental quotient) of 40, which was compatible with 4- to 5-month development. The physician (the author) felt the child might be deaf, but the audiologist felt that she reacted to sound when her hearing was tested. Because the child seemed so severely retarded, and because the mother had so many responsibilities with four other young children, the doctor recommended that the parents place Janet's name on a waiting list for admission to a state institution for the mentally retarded.

However, the parents absolutely refused to consider placement. They wanted to do everything they could to help Janet, and one of the suggestions of the physician was that they have another child. He told them that often a retarded child is stimulated by a younger brother or sister —they become good friends and have more in common than the older siblings do with the retarded child. He explained that often a younger sibling is able to help the retarded child develop in the areas of language and motor activities. The R.'s were concerned that they might have another retarded child, but they were assured by their obstetrician, pediatrician, and the author that there was absolutely no evidence that Janet's problem was hereditary. The parents were sufficiently reassured, and when Janet was two years old her brother was born. He was a normal, healthy boy, and was especially welcome in a family of five girls.

At the age of two years, Janet was definitely diagnosed as having cerebral palsy, and she began attending a cerebral palsy clinic. By the time she was three years old, she was able to hold her head straight, and the nystagmus had disappeared. However, both of these symptoms are still evident when she is very tired. In addition, she had learned to sit up by herself by the age of three, but she could not stand alone. The R.'s wondered if she would ever walk. At about that time, Janet's little brother began to walk, and Janet was determined that she would walk also. She began trying, even though her balance was poor. Her mother reported that for several months she looked like a battered child. She fell repeatedly and hit her head, requiring stitches so often that her parents kept a helmet on her in the daytime. She knocked out her front teeth, but her determination continued. She finally began making real progress when the hot summer weather arrived and her mother removed her stiff, high-topped shoes. Although the shoes had been prescribed by an orthopedist, and she was supposed to wear them at all times, she seemed able to keep her balance better when she was barefooted. She finally learned to take a few steps without falling.

When Janet was four years old, it was recommended that she attend a public school preschool class for the physically handicapped, which was part of the Crippled Children's Program in California. She was still not able to walk well, but at school she got around by carrying small sawhorses in each hand and moving them with her as she walked. The physical therapy which she had been having regularly at Childrens Hospital was continued at the school for the physically handicapped, as it was a part of the program at the school. Janet's teacher felt that she might be hard of hearing, and she was again tested by the audiologist, who again reported that her hearing was within normal limits. Janet still had no speech, and even though the audiologist and the specialist in mental retardation (the author) both assured the R.'s that Janet could hear, her teacher and her parents continued to feel that she might be hard of hearing.

When Janet was four and a half years old, Mrs. R. took her to the John Tracy Clinic, where her hearing was again tested. (The John Tracy Clinic was started by Mr. and Mrs. Spencer Tracy, whose son was deaf from birth. It has been invaluable to the parents of deaf children in Southern California.) The audiologist reported that she had a severe loss of hearing in one ear, and was totally deaf in the other. She was tested by the psychologist, who was experienced in working with children who were hard of hearing, and was found to be functioning up to the six-year-old level. Instead of being a mentally retarded child with mild cerebral palsy, she was a bright child with severe deafness and mild cerebral palsy!

Janet was fitted with a hearing aid so that she could take advantage of the hearing that she did have. Mrs. R. began to attend night classes at the John Tracy Clinic to learn how to work with a deaf child. The class met one night a week, and the parents learned to help their children. They also received counseling regarding the special problems relating to having a deaf child in the family.

Janet was still unable to walk alone, but at home she had a little table on wheels which she pushed ahead of her. When she was six years old, she found that she could stand alone. She began attending a public school for the physically handicapped, but her mother felt that she was not learning anything because the teachers had neither the training nor the equipment for teaching deaf children. Mrs. R. tried to make arrangements for Janet to attend a school for the deaf, but she soon found that though the Los Angeles schools have separate classes for the physically handicapped and special classes for the deaf, they do not have combination classes for the deaf and the physically handicapped.

It seemed obvious to everyone concerned that Janet's primary problem was her deafness, and that she would never learn in the school for the physically handicapped. However, it took a full-scale battle for the R.'s to convince the Board of Education, the special educators, and most of all, the principal of the school for the deaf that Janet should attend that school. The fear of the educators was that the child might hurt herself if she was in a facility which lacked the wheelchair ramps, the extra-wide doorways and the extra railings and other equipment at the school for the physically handicapped. Their fear of a lawsuit prohibited them from providing the education they knew the child needed. Finally, through sheer determination, the objections were worn away and it was agreed that Janet could attend the school for the deaf, but not before the R.'s were asked to sign a statement releasing the school from any responsibility in case of injury to the child while at school. Both Mr. and Mrs. R. knew this was an illegal and meaningless procedure, but it seemed to be the last face-saving effort of the administrators, so the R.'s signed the statement and Janet began attending the school for the deaf at the age of eight.

Each child at the school wore earphones which magnified the teacher's voice many times. Janet learned more about lip reading, in addition to the regular academic subjects. By this time, Janet's balance had improved to the point that she could walk, using tripod canes, and the following year she was able to walk without the canes. Also, when she was eight years old, her older sister taught her to swim, and swimming has become one of her favorite sports.

Janet attended the school for the deaf for five years.

She became a good lip reader, and began to develop speech. The R.'s also attribute her speech development to the fact that they were able to afford private speech therapy for her from the time she was nine years old until she was fourteen. This was expensive, as the sessions cost ten dollars an hour and were held once a week. This automatically prevents many children who really need speech therapy from receiving it. At the present time, Janet has braces on her teeth which interfere with the speech therapy exercises, but her parents hope she can have more speech therapy after the braces are removed.

Mrs. R. became very involved with the parents group at the school for the deaf, working closely with the principal, who had been afraid to have Janet in the school. Mrs. R. was instrumental in getting hot lunches delivered to the school, an accomplishment which required more determination and cutting of red tape. Later, when the school was being rebuilt, it was Mrs. R. who finally went to the Board of Education and saw to it that the children were removed from the campus during the construction. She rightly pointed out that the sounds of the hammers, power saws and other equipment were magnified many times by the earphones the children wore, and that the frequencies of those sounds could be especially damaging to whatever hearing the children had left. The children were bussed to a different location until the construction was finished.

During Janet's fifth year at the school for the deaf, Mrs. R. became increasingly concerned over the fact that she was not learning the academic subjects. At the end of the fifth year, when Janet was thirteen years old, she was doing work on the third-grade level. Mrs. R. felt that perhaps Janet's lip-reading ability was good enough for her to attend a school for normal children. The following year, Janet was enrolled in a Lutheran school a few blocks from her home. The teachers cooperated and made sure that she understood the assignments. She started out in a fifth-grade classroom, but she used textbooks from many different grade levels. For the first few weeks, she used a second-grade reader and a third-grade arithmetic book. But she seemed to love the challenge, and she absorbed knowledge like a sponge. Mrs. R. reported that she sat down with her books every day after school and studied until dinnertime, after which she went back to her books until bedtime. She enjoyed the studying so much that she did not care for television or games, and she made real progress.

The following year, she graduated from the Lutheran school, and her parents decided to try sending her to a junior high school for normal children. Even though there were still large gaps in Janet's knowledge and her reading comprehension was poor, they felt she should have a chance at the local junior high.

Again there was a battle, this time with the school doctor, who felt a deaf child should not be admitted to the school. Had the doctor known the determination and experience of the R.'s at overcoming obstacles, she might have given up before she started. Letters were written by Janet's former teachers at the Lutheran school, and there were conferences and meetings, before Janet was finally allowed to enroll in the school. She began attending regular classes, except for physical education. The task of competing in a much larger school was difficult and Janet was under a strain, but she enjoyed the social experience of going to regular junior high school. Mrs. R. sometimes despaired that she would be able to learn anything, and she worried that they had made a wrong decision in sending her to the school. Reading was especially difficult for her because of her limited vocabulary. Writing was also hard because of the vestiges of cerebral palsy, and it took her half an hour to write one side of one page of notebook paper. But in spite of the hard work, Janet loved going to the school. Although she was older than the other children, Janet had always been small of stature, and she was an attractive child. She thoroughly enjoyed the social contacts. Mrs. R. finally decided that whether or not she learned anything, the social experience of attending a normal school was reason enough for her to continue.

During Janet's second year at the school, Mrs. R. continued to feel that Janet was not really learning much academically, but when the day for the final report card came, she brought home one A, three B's and two C's!

Mrs. R. would like Janet to take typing next year and she plans to get her a typewriter to use at home. This should enable her to finish her homework much more easily. The R.'s are looking forward to having Janet graduate from junior high next year and continue on to regular high school.

Janet R. might well have ended up as a dull-eyed, lonely, forgotten child hidden away in a state hospital for the mentally retarded. Perhaps she would never have learned to walk. Perhaps no one would have discovered her deafness, and she would have become truly mentally retarded without the stimulation of anyone to care about her. As it is, she will become an attractive, fulfilled, contributing member of society.

Sometimes a child appears to be retarded because he has learning disabilities which may be due to sensory deprivation, emotional disturbances or defects in the central nervous system. Perceptual defects are the most common forms of specific learning disabilities. Such a handicap can be due to delayed maturation of the brain's ability to properly decipher symbols. In such a case, the child is unable to correctly interpret or reproduce written symbols.

These children sometimes visualize their letters as being upside down and backward. When they try to reproduce these symbols, they write them as they see them, upside down and backward. To such a child, learning to read and write is almost impossible.

Difficulties may also be caused by poor memory. Sometimes a child cannot keep a thought long enough to remember how a story has begun when he comes to the end. Other handicaps may be due to environmental deprivation. For example, a child may not understand words or phrases because he lacks the concepts they denote. He may also lack imagination and be unable to grasp any but concrete and present events.

The inability of these children to learn to read causes them to become frustrated and ashamed, and only compounds the problem. Ninety percent of the children with this disorder are boys. Fortunately, they usually improve with maturity and catch up by the age of sixteen or seventeen. Children with these handicaps may be referred to remedial reading programs in the public schools. These special programs can be very beneficial to them. Incidentally, some of the world's most brilliant thinkers appeared to have had perceptual handicaps. Tolstoy, James Watt, Isaac Newton and Winston Churchill all caused their families concern because of their late academic development.

Specific learning disabilities also occur in other academic subjects, such as arithmetic and spelling. It is of interest that Napoleon had difficulty with spelling and writing. Some children are also retarded in speech development, but with maturity they, too, improve. Charles Darwin had difficulty with language, and Albert Einstein was suspected of being mentally retarded as a small child because of his late speech development. He was unable to speak plainly even at the age of four.

Some children have speech defects due to organic

handicaps, such as a cleft palate. After surgical correction, these children can be helped by a speech therapist.

A more serious form of learning disability is dyslexia, or congenital word blindness. Children with this disorder have normal intelligence but cannot learn to read. They seem to lack some link in the chain of associations necessary for the complicated process of reading. To learn to read, a child must recognize the printed word and associate it with sound patterns which, in turn, are associated with meaning. For this chain of associations to occur, there must be correct visual and auditory perception, language, memory and thought.

Often children with reading difficulties lag in motor development and have poor eye–hand coordination. Physical education is usually helpful in conjunction with special reading programs. For the child with dyslexia, a correct diagnosis of the particular associations which are defective is important. Appropriate exercises are used to help alleviate the problem. For example, word-recognition drills are often used; phonics helps the child relate sounds to the printed syllables. Each child must be studied and treated as an individual. Often these children will continue throughout their lives to have difficulty in reading.

Another cause of pseudo-retardation is chronic disease in children. Some chronic diseases can cause children to be small in stature and can make them appear to be mentally retarded even though they have normal intelligence. Kidney disease and some forms of heart disease are such disorders. In addition, some children do not grow properly because of poor absorption of food, but they have normal intelligence. In essence, any chronic disease can make a child appear to be mentally retarded. Usually as these children grow older and as their disorders are kept under control, they become more normal in appearance.

There are so many children who may never
know what it's like to run and jump or
see the sky on a summer's day.

There are so many children who may never
hear a note of music, ride a bike, or
simply walk away—

There are so many children who will never
know what it's like to hear the wind in
the trees, the beat of the drums, or
what others might say.

For many of these children, the world is
lonely, abandoned,
Belonging to no one but themselves . . .
    They are left alone
    Out of another's ignorance and neglect.

Christine Koch

XII

Progress toward Normalization:

Care of the Mentally Handicapped Today in California

Traditionally, the care of handicapped persons has been developed through the efforts of lay groups organized for the benefit of the physically or mentally disabled. While the care of physically handicapped children has now become largely a pediatric responsibility, the care of the mentally retarded has too often been left to the psychiatrists, psychologists and social workers. The reason for this is that originally the mentally retarded and the mentally ill were lumped together in one group, since professionals were often unable to distinguish one from the other. The institutions for the mentally handicapped, which served both the mentally retarded and the mentally ill, were usually put under the jurisdiction of the psychiatric profession.

209

As scientific knowledge has advanced, it has become apparent that there are basic differences between the mentally retarded and the mentally ill, and that these differences require the skills of appropriate specialists. For example, the mentally ill are more often adults than children, while the mentally retarded are usually affected from birth. As children, the mentally retarded need the medical treatment which cannot be provided by someone in the psychiatric field, just as the psychiatric patient needs treatment which cannot be provided by a pediatrician.

In New York, Pennsylvania, Illinois, Texas and Ohio, the state institutions for the mentally retarded are still under the jurisdiction of psychiatrists, who are trained to care for the mentally ill rather than the retarded. This system probably developed because in the past, pediatricians seldom wished to become involved in the care of the mentally retarded in any measure beyond the usual procedures provided for any normal child. Today, however, services for the mentally retarded child are changing rapidly. The spectacular advances in chromosomal technology and biochemistry in the prevention and treatment of mental retardation in the last few years have changed the care of the retarded child into an exciting chapter in the ongoing progress of medicine. Today, we have the opportunity not only to correct the many physical handicaps of these patients but to participate in prevention programs which will either eliminate the occurrence of many forms of mental handicaps, or at least minimize the degree of mental retardation present in affected individuals.

Our system of medical care will have to change if we are to see a significant reduction in the occurrence of mental retardation. Unfortunately, we are not applying the scientific knowledge which we have to reduce the occurrence of mental retardation because bureaucratic change is involved. For example, although we know that common childhood diseases can and do have complications which cause mental retardation, in the State of California we have no agency designated and funded to make sure all children are immunized against diphtheria, tetanus, regular measles, polio and mumps. Our country, which had the technology to develop the polio, measles and German measles vaccines, has one of the lower rates of immunized children. The Scandinavian countries, through their system of medical care, have accomplished nearly 100 percent immunization of the children, but California data shows that only about fifty to seventy-five percent of our children are immunized against these preventable diseases.

Change is unsettling, even to those who consider it as progress. When change has an economic impact, you can rest assured it will be resisted by those affected adversely. There are many who say change cannot be legislated or imposed from above, but it is clear that both legislation and the hierarchy of the health care system must together develop a climate that encourages change, so that those working in the field of mental retardation can take advantage of scientific advances as they occur. While most members of the medical profession have been fairly active in instituting change within their own profession, they have not been effective at the legislative level in their respective states. If we are to move forward in the care of the handicapped in a constructive manner, we must develop more effective methods of encouraging legislative implementation of needed progress.

In each state, most of the tax dollars spent for the mentally retarded are utilized to staff and maintain institutions for their care. Often these institutions are located in rural settings where it is difficult to recruit staff and to institute training programs interacting with colleges and universities. In some states the programs in these institutions are deplorable. In a recent visit to Willowbrook State School on Staten Island, New York, a team of visitors saw 120 to 160 residents in locked wards with absolutely nothing to do. They were occupying two large day rooms, in each of which four attendants attempted to keep order. There were no towels or soap at the wash basins and no paper for the toilets. Some patients were naked and lying in their own excrement. The odor was stifling. It seemed as if one were transported back into the dark ages of despair. For this, the state of New York was paying $8,000 per patient per year for care! These conditions are typical of the average custodial institution, and according to Travis Thompson,* there are ninety-two thousand people living in such institutions in the United States today.

The rate of construction of state institutions, nationwide, is still significant, in spite of the fact that professionals already know that the traditional custodial institution is not a part of the normalization principle that we feel is right. Normalization refers to the process whereby mentally retarded persons are entitled to the same rights and privileges enjoyed by the "normal" populace. If a person becomes ill with cancer, he is not institutionalized in a locked ward somewhere out in the country! Perhaps this idea of isolating people with specific disorders is a vestige from the days of leper colonies and tuberculosis sanitariums. Before treatment was available for these contagious diseases, there was a logical reason for isolating them from contact with others, but there has never been a logical reason for the treatment which has been given the mentally retarded.

---

* *Behavior Modification of the Mentally Retarded* (Oxford University Press, 1972).

If we are truly committed to a principle such as normalization, then the first casualty in our present system would be the institution in its present form. And yet, our state governments are building more of them! Could it be that we don't really believe in this principle, and that we are merely giving lip service to it? The answer to this question is not simple. In California a decision was made by the state administration in 1972 to close all state institutions for the retarded and to work toward the development of community-based services by 1982. Unfortunately, very little planning had gone into preparing the public for such a move and there were not enough high-quality community facilities to meet the demand. While there are many advantages in having local community facilities for the care of the mentally retarded, perhaps there may always be a need for some small state institutions to care for the few profoundly retarded who are multiply-handicapped and need constant attention. In any event, the announcement of the plans seemed abrupt and uncompromising. The prospect of closure of all state institutions for the retarded mobilized two very powerful groups which forced the state to retreat from its decision. They were the parents of retarded persons in the institutions and the California State Employees Association. The parents felt very threatened by the idea that their retarded youngsters no longer would have the "protection" of the institution, and would be at "the mercy of the community." Regardless of the fact that the institutions were large and impersonal (about a thousand to two thousand residents) and most of them were located miles from their homes, the parents preferred them to the uncertainty of, as yet, nonexistent smaller facilities in their own communities. Parents who felt secure with their retarded child in a state institution feared they would again become responsible for him if he were placed in a local community setting.

Most parents found this totally unacceptable. And can anyone really blame them? Having a retarded child is difficult enough, but to have solved the problem by institutionalization, painful as that was, and now to be faced with the undoing of that decision was simply intolerable. Many vicious letters were sent to state legislators who thought they were doing the right thing in supporting the development of community services.

The role of the bureaucracy in self-perpetuation is also striking. In some states, employee associations have gone to court or threatened to strike when faced with alternatives to the traditional methods of care in the state institutions. The important factor has been the preservation of state jobs, and not what was best for the retarded person or his family. Callous as this may sound, it is absolutely true. There is something almost inherently evil in bigness. When organizations become so large that they lose sight of what is best for society, they begin to perpetuate the status quo to protect themselves. Thus the normalization principle faces two very determined opponents. Any state adopting this principle must be prepared for such opposition.

The movement toward normalization in California was begun in 1965, when Assemblyman Jerome Waldie introduced legislation authorizing the establishment of a regional center system funded by the state but operated by private, nonprofit organizations. The state legislature unanimously passed the bill (AB 691) to establish this regional center system, and included a novel feature in that funds were added to the operating budgets of the centers that permitted them to purchase services for parents who did not have enough money to carry out center recommendations. For example, if a retarded adult needs to participate in a day activity center, but his parents cannot afford the cost, the regional center will pay this amount for them.

If a retarded child needs dental care, this, too, can be paid for by the regional center if the parents cannot afford it. Other services which can be purchased by the regional center include physical therapy, a visiting nurse and many other services. Perhaps one of the most innovative services which can be purchased is respite care, in which the retarded child can be placed in a residential facility for a short period. This service is usually purchased if the mother becomes ill and cannot care for the child at home, or if the parents need a short relief from the complete responsibility of the child. Respite care is usually for a period of one or two weeks.

To date, twenty centers have been authorized with a state budget of $31,000,000 for 1975. They are to be located throughout California so that no family lives over two hours' drive from a center. Each center offers multidisciplinary diagnosis, evaluation and counseling. The centers serve all ages, and have been directed by the legislature to provide alternate solutions for parents whose retarded dependents require institutionalization. Thus the regional center can also purchase residential care in a private facility located near the child's home. There is no charge for diagnosis or counseling. If residential care is required, the family is assessed a monthly fee determined by its ability to pay. Under no circumstances is a family required to pay more than it would cost to keep a normal child at home. All financial obligation ceases when the retarded person has reached eighteen years of age.

The effectiveness of the centers in reducing admissions to state institutions has been dramatic. In 1969 there were 970 admissions to Pacific State Hospital in Los Angeles County, whereas in 1972 there were only 39. The state institutional population has dropped significantly from over 14,000 in 1965 to 10,000 in 1973. Similarly, the state had a waiting list for admission to its institutions of over 3,000 persons in 1965. Today, there is no waiting list at all. In fact, the institutions today have vacancies.

One might ask why California is trying to reduce the population of its institutions for the mentally retarded—after all, most of the residents cannot be independent, and their parents cannot be expected to provide a home for them all of their lives. A look at the problem, both past and present, will answer the question. The establishment of the institutions obviously grew out of a need. Some retarded persons are so disabled that it is very difficult to care for them at home. Many people were repelled by these profoundly retarded individuals. So institutions were established in isolated places where the retarded could be put away. For example, the state facility which serves San Francisco is in Sonoma, on the other side of the bay. Other large cities have carefully located their facilities for the retarded long distances away. Because of fear and ignorance on the part of the public and because of lack of medical knowledge, these institutions grew and prospered, taking in ever-larger populations of retarded individuals. Originally it was thought such people could not do anything, so no therapy or activity programs were established. The institutions became huge warehouses where retarded people lived out their lives. In recent years, advances in research have shown that most retarded persons can do many things, that they respond to attention and activity and therapy, and in fact, that some can fit into the normal population. Some good programs have been started in the institutions. However, most of them have grown so huge that they are overcrowded and usually understaffed and underfunded. They have been so inundated that they have simply been unable to make the needed changes.

Unfortunately, under the system followed in most

states, parents can commit their retarded child to a state institution, and there the child remains locked up for his lifetime. Many retarded persons are perfectly aware that it is their parents who are keeping them there. The reluctance of parents to take their retarded child out of the institution is understandable because they fear the responsibility of caring for him. Yet there is no logical reason for keeping retarded people imprisoned behind locked gates all of their lives; very few of them are threats to society. Only when there are facilities and programs for retarded people in their own communities can parents be expected to take them out of the state institutions. Most states do not have such facilities. California is fortunate in this respect. Since a special commission appointed by the governor in 1969 determined that many people were in state institutions for the retarded who did not actually belong there, the state has worked toward reduction of the state hospital populations. As a result, a variety of sheltered residential facilities for the retarded have been established in most communities. Other states should follow this lead if they wish to avoid building more of the huge prisons they call state institutions for the mentally retarded.

A recent development which has also contributed to the drop in population of the state institutions was the legislation enacted in 1972 giving the retarded adults the right to sign writs of habeas corpus if they wished to be released from the institutions. This innovative program is found in no state other than California. Under this program, any retarded adult who wishes to leave the institution may sign such a writ. After a writ has been signed, a representative of the regional center visits the applicant to determine whether or not he truly understands what his decision entails. This also gives the representative of the regional center an opportunity to observe the applicant firsthand

and get some idea as to whether he would do well outside the institution. Then a hearing is held before a judge, who must decide whether or not the individual will be allowed to leave the institution. Present for the hearing are the retarded person, his parents or guardians, a representative from the state hospital, and the representatives from the regional center.

The judge first verifies the fact that the retarded person wishes to leave the institution. He then questions the others present to determine whether the person would function well outside the institution and whether there are facilities available in the community to fill his needs. Most of these persons are obviously only mildly retarded. Others may be moderately retarded, but may feel that they would be happier in some sort of facility, such as a family-care home. Most of them want to be somewhere where they can have more privacy and more homelike surroundings than the impersonal atmosphere of the institution. Most of them also want to be someplace where they can work and, to some extent, earn a living. Recommendations are made by the representatives from the institution and the regional center before the judge makes his decision. Often parents oppose the idea because they feel more secure with their retarded adult offspring in the state institution. However, thus far, the only requests that have been refused are those of people who, it is felt, might be harmful to society if they were released. There are some mentally retarded homosexuals who are aggressive and could be a hazard to the safety of young children in the community. It is the consensus among professionals that these persons should remain in the institutions.

The retarded people who are placed in the community are sent either to board-and-care facilities, family-care homes or convalescent hospitals. A board-and-care facility is similar to a boarding house, in which each person has his own room and there is a central dining room. Whenever possible, these facilities are located near a sheltered workshop where the residents may be employed. Board-and-care facilities may have as few as ten residents or as many as fifty or sixty. The residents are not closely supervised and they are free to come and go as they wish. This type of placement is very appropriate for the mildly retarded.

A family-care arrangement is similar to foster-home care, in which the state pays a family to care for a small group of retarded people. Such a family receives $250 per month for each retarded person in its care. The people in these homes have fairly close supervision, as there are never more than six retarded residents in any one home. These homes are also often located near sheltered workshops. Since the family-care home provides closer supervision of the residents, it is more appropriate for the moderately retarded.

Occasionally, severely retarded persons are placed in community facilities, but since these people require constant supervision, they are placed in convalescent hospitals.

No person actually leaves the institution until a satisfactory facility has been found for him. The parents and the representative of the regional center usually work together to locate a residence which will be mutually acceptable. They take into consideration its proximity to their own home, the location of the nearest sheltered workshop or training center, and the physical appearance of the facility. Parents are encouraged to visit facilities before a choice is made so that they will be satisfied that their son or daughter is in good hands.

There are few statistics available on placements made in this manner because the use of the writ is such a recent development, but as of the present, only 5 percent of those released under this program have had to return to the state institution. Parents who were apprehensive about their adult offspring leaving the institution often seem pleased with the change. In nearly every case, it is easier for them to visit, and their son or daughter appears happier with the added independence.

With the decline in the number of residents in the California state institutions, the staffing ratio has improved, since the state has maintained the same number of staff members it had before the drop in the institutional populations. As a result, the programs in the institutions are somewhat of an improvement over the purely custodial care such as that described at Willowbrook in New York.

Today, some of the California institutions are becoming therapeutically oriented. A therapeutically oriented institution is one where the residents are given every opportunity to develop to their fullest potential. Such institutions have classes similar to the public school classes for the mentally retarded. They have sheltered workshops on the grounds for those residents who are capable of working. Some of them have programs that allow certain residents who have been trained for jobs to live at the institution but to go to work in the community each day. Pacific State Hospital in Pomona has such a program. These institutions provide physical therapy and speech therapy for those who need it. There are activity programs, such as dancing, singing and craft work, for those residents who are unable to take part in any educational program. There are also recreational activities, such as swimming and other sports, dances and parties. The residents are given the opportunity to participate in the Special Olympics, which are held at various places throughout the nation. This program, in which retarded children take part, was started in 1968 in Chicago by the Kennedy Foundation. A number of sports celebrities, including Rafer Johnson, Jerry West, Jesse Owens and Frank Gifford, have become involved in the Special Olympics and have helped coach the children. Behavior-shaping procedures are carried out which reward good behavior rather than punishing bad behavior. Thus the person who makes his bed neatly and picks up his clothes is allowed to go to the canteen to buy a Coke or go to the Saturday-night party. Although there are differences among the California institutions, they are all in a state of change, moving toward therapeutically oriented programs. Unfortunately, this is not true across the country—most institutions are still providing the same old custodial care.

As the programs in the state institutions in California improve, there will be increasing pressure upon regional center personnel to refer retarded persons to a state institution because it is better than a comparable community facility. To prevent this from happening, the state must be willing to spend an adequate amount of money on the retarded persons who are in community facilities so that they can have good services. For example, the state of California pays $250 a month or $3,000 a year for a retarded person to live in a family-care facility. If that same person were in a state institution, the cost to the state would be $12,000 a year. The state could pay a larger amount allowing the retarded person in the community to take part in more therapeutic programs and still not spend as much as it does for that person's care in a state institution. It seems clear that if the state government would put its major emphasis on purchasing community care for the retarded and insist on high standards for the services it buys, the retarded would be better served and the state would save money. And for the foreseeable future, the state should provide care for the profoundly retarded because of the lack of trained personnel in the community facilities. Ideally, it would seem that a combination of state and community-based programs is the answer to the complex problem of institution versus community facility.

Today we still have many diagnostic clinics which do not follow up on patients and thus only begin the process of evaluation. As we have gained experience in providing multidisciplinary services, we have realized that much professional time and effort are wasted because of the lack of implementation of recommendations. Evaluation is a long-term process. Diagnosis can often be made in a one-time examination, but treatment and rehabilitation must be accomplished over a period of months or years, and without this effort, evaluation remains inconclusive. For example, one quarter of the cases seen at the Child Development Clinic at Childrens Hospital of Los Angeles, after treatment and follow-up, were found to have been misdiagnosed or poorly evaluated. In most cases, the child had been thought to be more retarded than he actually was. This points up the importance of follow-up, since different recommendations can be made for appropriate remedial programs for the child. For example, a child thought to be severely retarded would not be referred to a public school program for the trainable retarded, but if a follow-up showed that he was only moderately retarded, he would be referred to such a program. More and more there will be units in medical centers which will provide follow-up services to those persons who are diagnosed and evaluated. California now has twenty such regional centers in which no case is closed unless death occurs. These units are providing services to persons of all ages, since mental retardation is a chronic condition which requires lifelong care. Therefore, the clinics which serve only retarded children will be expanding to serve adults as well. Another phase of these clinics is also disappearing. Until recently, there have been specialized clinics for mental retardation, cerebral palsy and epilepsy. These are now being combined under the designation of "developmental disabilities." This broadening of responsibility is a welcome development to both parents and professionals.

Today in the United States, a retarded child may be cared for in a variety of ways. The outdated practice of immediately "putting a child away" is seldom recommended any more, with the present trend being to consider each child as an individual. In California, when a physician knows or suspects that one of his patients is mentally retarded, he refers the parents to the nearest regional center, where the child is examined and evaluated. Any physical problems, such as hearing loss, poor eyesight or orthopedic disorders are dealt with as soon as possible.

If the child is found to be only mildly retarded, the parents will be counseled to keep the child at home. As he grows older, the parents may be advised to enroll him in a nursery school for normal children. When he reaches school age, he will be placed in a public school class for the educable retarded, where he will learn simple academic skills, as well as arts, crafts, music and physical education. If he is athletically inclined, he may even take part in the Special Olympics. Mildly retarded children can also usually participate in regular sports programs at school, making them feel more a part of the school. Such a child may attend public school through the twelfth grade, at which time he may seek employment. These young people may be referred to a State Vocational Rehabilitation Agency, where they can take part in training programs. In some special federal programs, they are paid while they learn.

Too often in the past, mildly retarded students, who were unable to compete in school, dropped out and took jobs mowing lawns or sweeping floors. Some of them got into trouble, as they were easily led astray, or wound up either in jail or on welfare. Actually three quarters of mildly retarded adults become productive citizens, and with recent improvements in education and training programs offered by the schools, this percentage should increase. A mildly retarded adult who has been taught a trade and who is socially acceptable in terms of cleanliness and good manners can nearly always secure employment and fit into the general population. Indeed, there are many mildly and moderately retarded individuals who can fill jobs in hotels and hospitals. They can also assist in laundries, plant nurseries and bakeries.

Employers who have given a chance to retarded workers report that there have been unexpected fringe benefits. The retarded employee is happy doing repetitive work which bores other workers. They stay longer on the job than the average employee, thus cutting down on turnover. After such an employee has learned a task, he faithfully carries it out without deviation. The foreman does not need to worry about the employee making independent decisions. Retarded workers have a low rate of absenteeism; when they learn a job, they take pride in it and seldom miss a day.

In the city of Los Angeles, there are 6,200 youngsters in the EMR (Educable Mentally Retarded) program. Recently the Los Angeles city schools, in cooperation with the National Association of Retarded Citizens and the federal government, has initiated an on-the-job training program for EMR youths. Employers who will employ and train a retarded young adult are reimbursed 50 percent of his salary for the first 160 hours worked and 25 percent for the second 160 hours worked, the only stipulation being that the employee be kept on if his work is satisfactory. The

McDonald's hamburger restaurants recently revealed that for the past two years they had taken advantage of this program and had employed a number of retarded youths to fry and assemble hamburgers. The project, which started on a trial basis, was very successful, and most of the other employees where the retarded individuals worked were not even aware that the cooks were retarded. Other firms in the Los Angeles area beginning to use retarded job trainees include International House of Pancakes, Ideal Brush Company of Van Nuys, the Los Angeles Hilton, the Seafood Tuna Company in San Pedro and the Bank of America's Data Processing Center.

A moderately retarded child today is usually kept at home. This is in contrast to what was done fifteen years ago. A 1957 study by Dr. Gerhart Saenger in New York revealed that 25 percent of the moderately retarded children died before reaching adulthood because many of them also have health problems such as heart disease or seizures. About half of them remained at home, and one quarter of them were in institutions. Actually the course of the moderately retarded child can follow that of the mildly retarded, except that he would not be able to fit into the school class for the educable retarded. He would, however, be able to function in the public school program for the trainable retarded child (TMR). In this program he would learn to keep himself clean and well-groomed. Some moderately retarded children do not even know how to dress themselves and are not toilet-trained when they start school. Usually they have difficulty handling knives and forks at mealtime. The teacher in the TMR class helps them learn good hygiene and basic good manners so that they can be socially acceptable. As the children grow older, they are usually taught some simple chores. The boys often learn to do gardening work and the girls are taught to make beds and do other housework. Children attend TMR classes for twelve years, and there is some effort being made to extend this so that a child may attend until the age of twenty-one.

These public school programs for the mildly and moderately retarded children are adapted to their intellectual capabilities. Usually the child whose IQ ranges between 50 and 70 is considered to be mildly retarded, and is placed in the EMR class. The child whose IQ is between 30 and 50 is considered moderately retarded, and is placed in the TMR class. However, since the IQ score is not always a reliable indication of a child's abilities, he may be switched to a more suitable program if he appears to be incorrectly placed. As a matter of fact, about 20 percent of the students in the TMR classes graduate into the EMR program.

Upon completion of the public school program for the trainable retarded, a moderately retarded youth is usually referred to a sheltered workshop where he can find employment. In addition, at age eighteen, the individual may apply to his local Social Welfare Department for Aid to the Totally Disabled (ATD). All parents should be aware that there are Social Security benefits available to most handicapped persons. They should check at their local office, especially when their child becomes eighteen. For such a person, ATD provides the basic living expenses plus a small amount of spending money each month. The amount provided for living expenses varies, depending upon what living arrangements are made. If the person continues to live in his own home, the amount is less than if he goes to a board-and-care facility or a foster home. In any case, the money for basic living expenses is sent directly to the person or agency providing room and board, while the monthly allowance goes directly to the retarded person. In addition, in California, retarded adults receiving ATD support are eligible for a work-training program which is both federally and state funded. Under this program, the fee is paid for the person to attend a sheltered workshop or an activity center. An activity center provides a program of singing, dancing and craft work which can be enjoyed by anyone, regardless of academic ability. If the moderately retarded adult is able to work productively in a sheltered workshop, he may do so; if he is unable to participate in this manner, he can still take part in the events at an activity center so that he can form friendships and have something meaningful to occupy his time.

A word should be said about the "normalization" of the moderately retarded. As has been stated, most mildly retarded people eventually fit in with the general population and become productive members of society. The moderately retarded are usually not able to do this. However, they should live as normal a life as possible. The authors feel it is important for such a person to leave home around the age of eighteen to twenty-one—after all, it is normal for a young person to leave home at this age. His parents will not always be there to look after him, and the retarded person should have the opportunity for a measure of independence. When a retarded adult remains at home, often his parents subconsciously infantilize him, or sometimes they use him as a sort of unpaid servant. By the time a retarded person has lived with his family for eighteen or twenty years, the parents have contributed to his upbringing as much as can reasonably be expected of them. His family will be more normal and he will be more normal if, like any other young adult, he goes to live in the community. Living on his own, he can go to work at a sheltered workshop or meet his friends at an activity center; he can go to the store for, say, an ice cream cone, and he can visit his family on holidays and special occasions.

The severely retarded child has an IQ ranging from

0 to 30. For the severely retarded person under twenty-one years of age, there are some public school facilities in California. California is one of the few states to provide an educational program for these children. This training takes place in developmental centers for the handicapped, where the severely retarded learn basic skills, such as feeding and toilet-training themselves, and self-discipline. There are not enough of these developmental centers to fill the need, but children who live at home get first preference. The severely retarded are those who are completely dependent all of their lives. Parents of these children should be aware that there is a high mortality rate among them, since they usually suffer from serious health problems, such as kidney disease, heart disease and skeletal abnormalities, including spina bifida. In a seventeen-year follow-up of severely retarded children done by Gerry Strickland and Richard Koch at Childrens Hospital in Los Angeles in 1973, it was found that 20 percent had died. Of those remaining, half were being cared for out of their homes. The other half were living at home but were in some sort of activity program.

The profoundly retarded, who also have a high mortality rate, are those children who have no measurable IQ. They never learn to walk or talk, and they are not aware of their environment. They often have difficulty swallowing and have poor cough reflexes. They have frequent bouts of pneumonia and diarrhea and often suffer from heart disease and kidney disease. The high mortality rate is understandable because of the associated health problems. The profoundly retarded are usually cared for in state institutions where they can have good medical care. In the seventeen-year follow-up conducted at Childrens Hospital in Los Angeles in 1973 it was found that 50 percent had died, and the rest were living at home. Probably the best hope for the profoundly retarded lies in the field of prevention.

It is important to integrate the mentally retarded into the normal community organizations at every opportunity. One sphere in which this can easily be accomplished is in the field of organized religion; if there is any organization within the community which should be accepting and understanding of the problems of the retarded, it is the Church. A child need not read or write to participate in the fellowship and mutual concern which should be a part of any church family or congregation. Indeed, often the retarded can accept on faith those concepts which the person who demands scientific facts finds difficult to believe. Many retarded children have special musical and artistic talents, and can participate in a meaningful way in the junior choir and the arts and crafts activities of the church school. Retarded adults can also feel useful and needed in such capacities.

Increasingly, churches and synagogues are establishing daily nursery schools as part of the church program. These nursery schools should make special efforts to include retarded children and minority children in their enrollment. This not only would benefit the retarded children, but would also aid the others in becoming more accepting of individual differences among people. If children can interact on a daily basis with the retarded as well as the normal, the Oriental and Black as well as the white, perhaps they will not fall prey to the bigotry and racism which are two of the worst communicable diseases of our time.

All children need to be loved,
And all children want to give love—

For love far surpasses all material possessions,
   And through love, children grow—
Spiritually, mentally and physically.

Love is the ultimate catalyst to bring about
   change in our world
For *all* the children of tomorrow!

Christine Koch

XIII

Sex and the Mentally Retarded

Perhaps one of the main reasons we have isolated retarded people behind locked gates is because we have sexual fears. The parents of a retarded girl are often worried, especially as she grows older, that she will be taken advantage of if she is not under close supervision. Parents of retarded boys may be fearful that their sons will be attracted sexually to girls in the neighborhood. And, no doubt, parents of normal girls are fearful that the retarded boy around the corner may attack their daughters. So we have solved the problem by locking up the retarded and attempting to keep them supervised so that no sexual contact can take place between the males and females.

Actually, the attempt of the institutions to enforce

231

celibacy among the residents has not been completely successful; pregnancies occur occasionally. In addition, because of the difficulty in obtaining qualified staff personnel, untrustworthy persons are occasionally hired who take sexual advantage of the residents. Usually when a pregnancy occurs, the parents of the woman are consulted as to what should be done. They almost invariably decide on abortion. This is probably wise, since a retarded woman might well bear a retarded child, especially if she is moderately or severely retarded. If the woman is under eighteen years of age the parents can make the decision themselves. If she is over eighteen she is considered to be an adult, and her written consent is required; a doctor would explain the problem to her, and in most cases, it is possible to make her understand that she is going to have a baby who might very well be retarded as she is. Retarded people realize that they are different, and they usually feel inadequate in coping with difficult situations. They seldom have any desire to bear a child who might be mentally retarded; they can also usually see how difficult it would be for them to care for a baby. If it is felt that the woman understands the problem and understands the proposed operation, and if she agrees to have it done she is asked to sign a consent statement. However, if she is too retarded to understand the situation or the explanation, a court order must be obtained before the abortion is performed. This can be done by contacting a lawyer or a district attorney, who starts the legal procedure.

Profoundly retarded women usually have no interest in sex, and do not become pregnant unless they are raped.

Another problem in the institutions is masturbation. This is especially true in the older custodial-type of facilities where there are absolutely no activities for the residents. It is very natural that if a hundred and fifty moderately and severely retarded persons are herded into a day room where there are no toys, no pictures or furniture, and where there are only two attendants to keep order, masturbation would be the order of the day. In many of these institutions, the residents are never taken outside for a walk or a picnic; they never have any craft projects or sports activities. So they spend day after day in the same bare room masturbating. What else can we expect?

With the recent trend toward normalization and away from institutional care for the retarded, we are again faced with the problem of sex and the mentally retarded because most mentally retarded persons have very normal sex urges and desires. It is only the very severely and the profoundly retarded who have no interest in sex. Just as we are finding that many retarded people can function quite well in the community if they have the training to make them socially acceptable, we are finding that their sex drives can be satisfied in acceptable ways.

In the therapy-oriented institutions, where there are many activity programs for the residents, the problem of masturbation and sexual promiscuity is not as pronounced as it is in the custodial institutions. The residents can work off some of their sexual energy by participating in sports activities. Arts and crafts can occupy time which might otherwise be spent masturbating. Folk dancing and choral singing give the residents the opportunity to have meaningful associations with people of the opposite sex. Picnics, parties and dances are a regular part of the program in some institutions. In these institutions, resident couples do sometimes form relationships of mutual love and respect. However, there has never been any way for these couples to consummate their feeling for each other, except in some clandestine moments when they can escape the vigilant eye of the supervisory personnel. One solution would be the construction of apartments for married residents; this would create a much healthier atmosphere than the present arrangement. Sweden has had such facilities for retarded couples for some time. Some private nonprofit organizations in California have started similar programs, but this innovation is not yet widely seen in the United States.

As already mentioned, in California many of the retarded people are now leaving the institutions and going to live in the community, either in board-and-care residences or in family-care homes. There is no reason why board-and-care facilities could not have small apartments or suites of rooms for retarded couples.

Of course, one legitimate objection to the idea of allowing the mentally retarded to have heterosexual relations is the fear that they will produce children whom they will be unable to care for and who might also be mentally retarded. Just as normal people are encouraged to have counseling when they are considering marriage, retarded people should also be given this opportunity. Most retarded people are very much aware of the motives of other people. They sense whether or not a person is sincere or just making fun of them. They realize that they are different and have special problems. They are usually very grateful when a person will listen to their problems and concerns, and offer some helpful advice. The retarded person who is contemplating marriage is usually as concerned as those around him about the ramifications of such a move. Therefore, marriage counseling is both appropriate and workable for the mentally retarded. Most retarded people can understand when it is explained to them that it would be very difficult for them to raise children; they can also understand that their children might be like them. Often, the male will decide to have himself sterilized. When retarded people realize that there are ways of preventing pregnancy, and when they are counseled understandingly, they usually respond in a responsible manner.

Parents often worry because their retarded child seems sexually promiscuous. This is especially true of some mildly retarded girls. Some of them are eager to have sex at any and all opportunities. Indeed, some retarded girls are very affectionate and occasionally boys are aggressive. The parents sometimes decide that the best solution is to have their child sterilized. At one time, sterilization was done routinely in many institutions for the retarded, but this is no longer the case. If a child is under eighteen years of age, the parents usually need a court order for the sterilization. If the retarded person is over eighteen, he must give his written consent. And if a person is agreeable to the procedure but is unable to sign his name, he can mark an X.

Sterilization would be inappropriate for the mildly retarded, since these people usually become part of the general population as adults. They can nearly always hold jobs and often they can raise families. They would be counseled to have no more than one or two children, since they are usually not capable of earning much money. It is also true that a mildly retarded couple runs a higher risk of having a retarded child than the average couple. A mildly retarded woman can successfully use the pill if she is reliable. If the pill presents problems for her, she can use the IUD (intrauterine device, or plastic loop), which is inserted through the vagina into the mouth of the uterus by the doctor. The advantage of this type of birth control for a retarded woman is that she does not have to worry about taking a pill on schedule. The IUD is painless and it is 90 percent effective in protecting against conception. The woman becomes fertile again when the IUD is removed. Of course, after a mildly retarded couple have had one or two children, the husband can have a vasectomy (sterilization) and end the worry of further pregnancies. This operation, done under local anesthetic, is relatively painless, and it takes about ten minutes in a urologist's office. Some men are under the impression that they cannot enjoy the sex act after they have had a vasectomy. This is not true. It should be explained to retarded men that this operation does not interfere with sexual satisfaction.

As in other phases of a retarded child's activities, it is important for parents to teach appropriate social behavior in sex-related activities. The importance of appropriate behavior is often overlooked by parents as well as professionals. The child who clings to the stranger with excessive affection or while drooling, the adolescent who is noisy and boisterous, the adult with obscene gesturing all cause the public to reject the retarded person.

Sexual outlets are important to teach retarded teenagers and adults. Masturbation in public is a problem usually caused by the fact that the parents have not taught the individual that certain activities are appropriate in the bathroom or bedroom, but not in the living room or the front yard. If retarded people are not taught the proper place to release their sex urges, they engage in activities which are misunderstood by the public and which often get them into trouble with the law.

Recently the author saw a twenty-seven-year-old retarded man in the Los Angeles County jail who had been in various penal facilities in California for three and a half years. He had been charged with child molestation. He had a documented IQ of 36, and had been living at home until he committed the offense. He was not involved in any activity programs and spent his time wandering the streets. One day, he accosted a 7-year-old girl and told her to lie down on the street. Then he lay on top of her. She began to scream and neighbors immediately apprehended the retarded man. The police came and he was taken to court, where he was sentenced as a mentally disordered sex offender. Subsequently he was admitted to the State Hospital for Sex

Offenders at Atascadero, California, where he remained for two years before it was decided that he was inappropriately placed. He was then referred back to jail so that his case could be reviewed by the courts and charges against him dismissed. This one simple error in behavior caused this retarded person three and a half years of incarceration. Actually what this person needed was some counseling. No one had ever told him that such behavior was not appropriate; no one had ever told him what caused him to have an erection. Some moderately retarded persons must even be taught to release their sexual urges through masturbation. If this youth had been in some sort of activity program, he probably would not have gotten involved with the law. He will probably go back home, but now he will have counseling sessions with a doctor. The parents will also have some counseling with a social worker so that they can learn better techniques of supervision. His parents are anxious to have him back. They feel that he is really a harmless individual who did not actually know what he was doing or why he was doing it. The police and the courts are becoming more aware of the problems and the rights of the mentally retarded, but cases such as this are not too uncommon.

Although we have very little experience with marriage for the mentally retarded here in the United States, and some states even have laws prohibiting it, the trend to allow such marriage is healthy and should be encouraged.

XIV
Unproven Treatments for Mental Retardation

In seeking help for their mentally retarded children, parents are sometimes tempted to turn to treatments which seem to hold promise of beneficial results but which are not approved by established medical specialists. Parents are sometimes confused, and understandably so. It seems strange to them that their child's doctor would not be enthusiastic about any therapy that might help their child. The developers of special treatments and medications often publicize testimonials and case histories of people who have either been cured of mental retardation or benefited greatly from the treatments. It is also disturbing to parents that the developers of some treatments are prevented by the Food and Drug Administration (FDA) from selling their products across state lines, and that some of these products are completely banned in the United States. The fact that these therapies are often available in other countries, such as Switzerland and Mexico, also seems unfathomable. "Why is it," a parent will ask, "that I cannot buy a medication in this country, which has alleviated symptoms, and in some cases, cured mental retardation?"

Actually, there is a psychosomatic factor in many illnesses, and people are often helped by treatment which is of no medicinal value. Often children do actually improve when certain therapies are used, not so much because of the therapy itself but because of the added attention the child gets, and the expectations of the parents that the child will improve.

In order to give its official approval, the FDA must have scientific proof beyond testimonials and case histories. And although people sometimes become impatient with the FDA and its exacting studies of medications, we should be thankful for the protection it affords us. If it had not been for the vigilance of the FDA, the drug thalidomide would have been sold in this country and thousands of children would have had tragic deformities before the cause was discovered.

To determine the value of a medication, the FDA requires scientific proof such as a double blind study showing beyond any doubt that the therapy accomplishes the beneficial results claimed by the manufacturer. The following is an example of the double blind study.

The author was involved in a study of the effects of thyroid hormone on Down's syndrome babies. Although thyroid hormone is not a controversial or dangerous drug, there was uncertainty as to whether it was of value in the treatment of Down's syndrome. Some doctors felt that thyroid was very helpful to Down's syndrome children, and that it actually improved their IQ. For the double blind study, a group of Down's syndrome babies were examined by two doctors to make sure that they did indeed have the disorder. The study could have been misleading if those participating did not actually have it. Occasionally a hypothyroid person resembles an individual with Down's syndrome, so it was vitally important that those participating in the study be properly diagnosed. The babies were also examined and tested by a psychologist to determine their developmental quotient. They were then divided at random by the person who was to dispense the medication. Half of the group was put on a dosage of thyroid extract daily, while the other half was put on a daily dosage of a placebo. (A placebo is a harmless substance of no medicinal value, usually sugar or chalk.) Neither the doctors and the psychologist nor the parents of the patients knew which infants were receiving the thyroid extract and which were receiving the placebo, since the pills were made to look identical. Only the person dispensing the medication kept a record of which patients actually received the hormone. Because of this, the parents of the children receiving the placebo were as enthusiastic and hopeful about the treatment as the parents of the children receiving the medication. The children all received extra attention. They were given their medicine, which was supposed to help them. Every three to six months they were brought to the hospital for special examinations to see what progress they had made. They were weighed, measured and given physical examinations. Once a year, psychological evaluations were done on the children. Careful records were kept. The study lasted three years. As the study progressed, the doctors speculated as to which patients were receiving the placebo and which were receiving the thyroid extract. Some of the babies made significant progress. One child walked at the age of fifteen months. The average age of walking for a Down's syndrome child is twenty-seven months. Another started saying words at eighteen months. The average age of talking for a Down's syndrome child is two and a half to three years. Another child sat up by himself at seven months, rather than the usual age of nine months. The doctors were nearly convinced that the children making the most progress were those who were receiving thyroid extract. However, at the end of the study, it was found that some of the children who had made the most progress were those who had been taking the placebo. Some of the children taking thyroid had also made good progress. Thus, the finding of the study was that the use of thyroid for Down's syndrome children has no significant effect on their progress, and the only Down's syndrome children who should take thyroid are those who actually have a thyroid deficiency.

This research was called a double blind study because neither the doctors nor the patients knew which patients were receiving the placebo and which were receiving the actual medication. In such a study, the results have been scientifically proven. This is far different from the data gathered when a doctor gives a patient a medication he feels will be helpful. He tells the parents that he feels the child will improve, and in many cases the child will live up to expectations and will indeed show improvement. In such a case it is impossible to know whether the medication caused the improvement or whether the added attention and expectation for improvement had a placebo effect. Those developers of medications who will not submit the therapy to the proof of a double blind study of sufficient proportions to provide sound scientific data and who provide "proof" only in terms of case histories and success testimonials often take advantage of people by charging high fees. In some cases the treatments are actually detrimental to the well-being of the patient. For example, a child with a brain tumor may begin to lose the use of his arms and legs. There have been cases where such a child has been taken to a chiropractor for treatment. While chiropractors can sometimes help people with strained backs, they do not have the training to treat a brain tumor. The time lost in such a case—while the child is given spinal adjustments to alleviate the symptoms and while the brain tumor continues to grow—can make the difference between life and death to the child.

The cult of chiropractics was begun some seventy-seven years ago by Daniel Palmer, a grocer, fish peddler, and magnetic healer. Palmer was said to have cured a man's deafness with a well-aimed whack on the back. He subsequently started the Palmer method of chiropractics. Basic to this type of treatment is the belief that most diseases and illnesses are caused by spinal subluxations (vertebrae which have slipped out of alignment). According to this theory, these illnesses can be treated and cured by spinal adjustment and manipulation. No scientific evidence was ever offered by Palmer to substantiate his theory, but many people felt that they were helped by his treatments. It is possible that chiropractics may be somewhat akin to the newly rediscovered practice of acupuncture. Actually, scientists have never fully understood the development and complexity of the nervous system. Acupuncturists have learned that they can usually relieve pain by inserting needles to stimulate certain nerve centers. Perhaps, in like manner, chiropractors have developed methods of relieving pain by manually stimulating some of these same nerve centers. This whole field of nerve stimulation is belatedly receiving scientific attention and study.

There are honest and sincere chiropractors, who truly

feel that they can help patients with certain types of disorders, but unfortunately, there are some unscrupulous practitioners who have attempted to cure mental retardation by administering spinal adjustments. Such treatments do not cure mental retardation, and sometimes delay needed therapy.

There are other unproven treatments that are used to treat brain-damaged persons. One such treatment has patterning as its basic technique. The developers of this form of treatment feel that the basic reason for physical and mental retardation is that certain children either skipped an early phase of their motor development or did not develop correct patterns in movement. The treatment consists of having the patient lie on the floor while his arms, legs and head are moved in swimming or crawling patterns. This procedure is carried out four times a day for five minutes at a time, seven days a week. The patterning movements are so complex and time-consuming, and the other procedures which are a part of the treatment so exacting, that usually the parents alone cannot possibly keep up the schedule, and neighbors and friends must help. Sometimes a hundred to two hundred volunteers per week are required to carry out the treatment. The developers of this therapy have the theory that the patterning of the extremities in correct swimming and crawling movements will stimulate the growth of healthy brain cells to take over the function from defective ones. They also place emphasis on the hemispheric dominance of the brain. If the left side, or left hemisphere, of the brain is dominant, a person is right-handed, and if a person is left-handed the right side of the brain is said to be dominant. In other words, if a person is right-handed, the electrical impulse which initiates motor activity comes from the left side of the brain and vice versa. People who are ambidextrous have not established a hemispheric dominance. Some brain-damaged individuals are ambidextrous, but some very bright people are also ambidextrous and no controlled study has ever given scientific proof that ambidexterity is a sign of brain damage. However, in this treatment, the establishment of dominance is considered to be important, and children are sometimes restricted to the use of one hand or one eye in an effort to bring about this dominance. In addition, the technique of masking is sometimes used, in which the patient breathes into a bag or plastic mask for thirty to sixty seconds out of each waking hour. This is another procedure that has not been proven in a controlled study. The theory is that the air in the bag which has a high carbon dioxide content will stimulate a greater flow of blood to the brain. Children are also given eye exercises and reading exercises at a very early age, usually at about two years.

Actually, movements similar to the patterning techniques are often used by physical therapists in training stroke or cerebral palsy patients to have better control of their arms and legs, and the patterning therapy began as a treatment for cerebral palsy patients. It has merely been expanded by its developers as a treatment for most forms of brain damage. There is no rational basis for believing that because a certain treatment can help a person with cerebral palsy, it can help a person with mental retardation. And yet, this is the basic theory of the patterning treatment.

In patterning, special significance is attached to regular and absolute compliance with all of the instructions. Most families find the procedure so exacting that it is almost impossible to follow all the instructions without some slight deviation. If a child does not show improvement, it can be argued that the treatment had not been carried out correctly by the parents or that occasionally patterning sessions were missed or were not done on schedule.

Although this treatment could easily be tested so that

objective scientific proof of the claimed benefits could be obtained, no such successful study has been forthcoming. This could be accomplished by studying a group of persons with a specific type of brain damage, such as those suffering the symptoms of anoxia at birth. The group could then be divided, with half of the patients being treated by patterning techniques and the other half by the conventional methods of physical therapy, good nutrition and good home care. Over a period of three years, records of such a study could provide reliable scientific proof regarding the effectiveness of patterning as a treatment. Until such a study is done, this form of treatment remains a questionable type of therapy.*

Another treatment which has been difficult to evaluate is the U series of drugs, which is used in Detroit for the treatment of Down's syndrome. The U series consists of a combination of about fifty medications, including vitamins, minerals, hormones, enzymes and glutamic acid (an amino acid). Although the developer of this treatment claims that it can improve the physical and mental condition of Down's syndrome children, he has offered no conclusive scientific proof. Only one double blind study has been carried out with this medication, and it showed that the U series was of no proven value in the treatment of Down's syndrome. While there is no scientific proof that the U series is effective in improving Down's syndrome patients, there is no proof that it is harmful; therefore it is available in Michigan, where it was developed. However, before permitting interstate shipment of a product, the FDA must have scien-

---

* In 1968 the American Academy of Pediatrics published a statement questioning the effectiveness of this form of treatment. The statement can be found in the May issue of the *Journal of Pediatrics*, Vol. 72, p. 750, or it can be obtained without charge by writing the American Academy of Pediatrics, P.O. Box 1034, Evanston, Ill. 60204.

tific proof that it accomplishes the beneficial effects claimed for it; because of this requirement the U series has not been approved for interstate shipment. Many parents, searching for aid for their Down's syndrome children, have traveled to Detroit and have spent huge amounts of money for the U series. And some of the patients have indeed improved. However, many physicians in the field of mental retardation have not been able to document any real benefit from the U series when they have evaluated patients who have undergone this treatment. The authors feel that the developer of this treatment is very sincere in his belief that he can actually alleviate the symptoms of Down's syndrome and that the children he treats do improve in their intellectual functioning. In our opinion, however, the improvement that he has recorded can be accomplished with any Down's syndrome child receiving good nutrition and good home care, and is unrelated to the drug therapy. As with the placebo, the child receives added attention. The doctor is kind and interested in the problem; he feels confident his treatment can help. The parents are encouraged and take special notice of the child's activities. It is little wonder that the child does indeed improve.

Another treatment, developed some years ago in Switzerland, is known as cellular therapy. This treatment has been used for numerous diseases, including mental retardation. The basic theory here is that certain organs of the body can be revitalized by injections prepared from the corresponding organs of embryos taken from freshly killed animals. According to the theory, a person with liver disease would receive injections of embryonic liver cells, and one with mental retardation would receive injections of embryonic brain cells, and so on. To date, no publications have appeared in the American pediatric literature showing conclusive benefit derived from this therapy. However, many conscientious parents have taken their children to Zurich for the treatment at great expense. Understandably, they wanted to leave no stone unturned in their efforts to help their children. Perhaps if doctors showed more interest and took time to establish a relationship of trust between the parents of retarded patients and themselves, the parents would not be so inclined to try unproven treatments that offer no realistic basis for hope. If parents feel that their doctor is not really interested in their child; if he says he knows of no treatment for him, it is only natural for them to seek help from someone else.

From time to time certain fads develop in the treatment of mental retardation. About twenty years ago, many doctors treated their mentally retarded patients with glutamic acid, which is a constituent of all protein. This substance was thought to be important in brain-cell metabolism and would raise the IQ of the patients. Although subsequent controlled studies have been done, not one has proven that it is of any value in the treatment of mental retardation. Yet it is still widely used in South America.

Another substance which was thought to be of benefit to mentally retarded children with Down's syndrome was a chemical called 5-hydroxytryptophane. This substance is converted to serotonin by the body, a substance used in brain-cell metabolism. It was found that Down's syndrome children had a low level of serotonin in their blood, and 5-hydroxytryptophane was given to raise the serotonin level in the hope that it would improve the intellectual functioning. However, a double blind study of 5-hydroxytryptophane was conducted between 1970 and 1973 by Dr. Mary Coleman, and she found this treatment to be of no value.

Lastly, a few words should be said about the use of food supplements, vitamins and minerals. One of the newest therapies for numerous disorders is the use of megavitamin dosages; this consists of administering many times the daily requirement of a specific vitamin. For example, many people are taking massive dosages of vitamin E, which is said to rejuvenate aging tissues. Megavitamins have also been tried in the treatment of mental retardation and of schizophrenia, but they have proven to be of no value. True, there are some diseases causing mental retardation in which huge vitamin dosages are indicated. In methyl-malonicaciduria, for example, the body is unable to properly use vitamin B_{12}, and therefore this vitamin must be given in massive dosages. Some people assume that if huge amounts of vitamin B_{12} help the patient with methyl-malonicaciduria, they will also help the patient with Down's syndrome or learning disorders. This is not true, and parents should consult a doctor before dosing themselves or their children with enormous amounts of vitamins.

It is unfortunate that there are unscrupulous practitioners who prey upon people who have certain problems that still defy medical science. This probably occurs more often in the fields of therapy for cancer and for mental retardation than in any other areas. Before embarking on any special therapy, parents should consult their family doctor or pediatrician. He has access to the latest professional journals, and would know of any new, reliable treatment. Oftentimes parents are hesitant to discuss such a decision with their doctor, thinking that he might misunderstand. Any legitimate physician should be understanding of the desire of parents to do everything possible to help their child and should be willing to take the time to explain the basic theory of the treatment they are considering, as well as the scientific facts regarding the therapy. If it is a treatment which has proven to be of no value, he should let them know this; if it is a treatment he considers potentially harmful, he should certainly warn them. But he should not try to make a decision for them; parents should be told that occasionally unproven treatments do produce some improvement and they are certainly free to do as they wish with their child. He should put them at ease by emphasizing that if they ever wish to return, he will be happy to treat their child again. Parents should be suspicious of any treatment not accepted by the American Medical Association and banned by the Food and Drug Administration. It is often helpful for parents to inquire at the local Association for Retarded Citizens, the County Health Department, the local medical society or the public school to locate the proper resources. If parents have questions about the validity of any specific treatment, they can write the Department of Investigation, American Medical Association, 535 N. Dearborn St., Chicago, Ill. 70610. This organization will furnish information upon all inquiries. They might also wish to send for the pamphlet *The ABC's of Quackery and Sound Medical Care*, by writing to the National Association for Retarded Citizens, 2709 Ave. E East, P.O. Box 6109, Arlington, Texas 76011.

XV
Guardianship

A nagging worry for the parents of a retarded person has always been what would happen to the retarded child should he outlive them. This is a very real problem because today most retarded individuals do outlive their parents.

In California this problem is solved by the use of guardians, conservators and advisers. Retarded persons have legal civil rights and many of them can make contracts, but since they usually need varying degrees of advice and assistance, it is important for parents of retarded children to make these arrangements when the child reaches the age of eighteen.

Each of these classifications carries somewhat different responsibilities. The California Department of Health lists them as follows:

A *guardian* is a person appointed to take care of the person and property, or person or property of another. The latter person is called the *ward* of the guardian. The relationship of guardian and ward is confidential and is subject to the provisions of law relating to trusts. In the management and disposition of the person or property committed to him, a guardian may be regulated and controlled by the court.

A *conservator* is a person appointed to take care of the person and property, or person or property of a *conservatee*. Conservatorship may be used instead of guardianship, when there is an objection to the use of the word "guardian," or if the disability is temporary. Since conservatorship proceedings normally do not involve a finding of incompetence, in any cases of actual incompetence, guardianship is recommended.

An *adviser* provides advice and guidance to a mentally retarded person, and is not appointed by a court. The provision for such services is not dependent upon a finding of incompetency, nor does it abrogate any civil rights otherwise possessed by the mentally retarded person.

Guardianship is a legal procedure in which a person must be adjudicated incompetent. According to the state Probate Code, a person is mentally incompetent when he is "unable, unassisted, properly to manage and take care of himself or his property, and by reason thereof is likely to be deceived or imposed upon by artful or designing persons." Guardianship and conservatorship are very similar except that conservatorship does not involve a finding of mental incompetency. The responsibilities of a guardian or conservator are to make certain that the ward is properly fed, housed and clothed, and that his medical care needs are met. It is also the responsibility of the guardian or conservator to see that the ward's rights are implemented and that opportunities are made available to him so that he achieves his optimum potential.

California is one of the few states that have conservators, and it is the only state to have advisers. All of the states provide for the appointment of guardians who protect the rights of their wards. The present trend in California is to use guardians for all but the mildly retarded. A conservator offers a mildly retarded person the same type of protection as does a guardian, the only difference being that when a conservator is appointed it is not necessary that the ward be found incompetent.

The regional center aids families in initiating the legal procedure involved in guardianship appointment. Usually parents wish to nominate themselves as guardians. In such a case, the parents would contact an attorney to draw up the proper papers and, in writing, nominate themselves to be legal guardians or conservators. They would document that their child needed a legal guardian or conservator for himself and/or his estate. If they were nominating themselves as guardians, they would have to secure a certificate from a licensed physician as to the mental incompetency of the child. To ensure that the child would have continuing care, the parents might also name a person to be nominated upon their death. This person can be named in any written document, such as a will or letter, and can be any person the parents might wish, such as a family friend, a sibling or other relative of the retarded person, or in the absence of any qualified person, it could be the director of the state Department of Health. A copy of that portion of the document would be dated and sent to the regional center serving the area where the mentally retarded individual lives, and would become a part of the regional center case record, along with a medical and social summary and an ongoing plan for the person.

When all of the relevant material has been assembled

and all persons involved (siblings of the mentally retarded person, other close relatives, etc.) have been notified, a hearing is held in superior court and the court makes the appointment of the guardian or conservator. In attendance at the hearing are the parents, their attorney, often the retarded person and anyone else involved.

At the death of the parents, another hearing is scheduled regarding the appointment of the person nominated by the parents to take over under these conditions.

If the director of the Health Department had been nominated by the parents, the regional center would have so notified the Bureau of Developmental Disabilities, with the recommendation that the director accept the nomination. Again, all relevant records would be assembled and all concerned people notified, and another hearing would be held in which the director would be appointed. If he is named, the regional center acts as the guardian for the life of the individual or until such time as the person no longer needs a guardian. An annual report is made by the regional center to the Bureau of Developmental Disabilities as to the situation of the retarded individual.

The role of the adviser, or citizen advocate, deserves more discussion. Such a person can fulfill a crying need for a retarded person. Too often, retarded individuals exist in institutions or facilities where, though they are fed and clothed, there is no personal concern for their needs and desires. Their lives are lonely and barren of companionship. The citizen advocate is a person who makes a commitment to provide personal concern and guidance on a one-to-one basis—the kind of concern and guidance one's own family would provide. A citizen advocate might take his ward shopping for clothes, help him obtain a driver's license, help prepare his tax returns or start a bank account. The retarded person could look forward to phone calls, letters and visits from such a person.

Some teenage clubs are already taking part in projects in which the members work personally with retarded youths of their age. They plan dances and parties for the retarded teenagers of their community. With the present trend toward early retirement and more leisure time, this is a most worthwhile project for retired people and senior citizens as well. It requires time and dedication, but it can be very rewarding.

Guardianship is obviously for the protection of the mentally retarded ward. Since a finding of mental incompetence limits the activities in which a person may legally participate, the problem of guaranteeing the civil rights of the retarded person becomes difficult. The legal rights of the mentally retarded are very poorly understood by most people, and the laws of most states concerning people who have been adjudicated incompetent are a hodge-podge of antiquated terms and ambiguity.

The following examination of the effect of guardianship on the civil rights of the mentally retarded person in California was prepared by the California Association for the Retarded. Since guardianship serves primarily a protective purpose, it is designed to take from the ward the legal capacity to engage in certain activities that would endanger his safety or financial security. The problem presented by the guardianship legislation of most states is to determine which activities the ward is legally incapable of performing; too often the adjudication of incompetence which follows the appointment of a guardian impairs the legal capacity of the ward to exercise his basic civil rights. The legal capacity vested in the mentally retarded person under guardianship should reflect as accurately as possible the *actual* competency of that person.

If a retarded person has been placed under a guardian and therefore has been declared legally incompetent, does he have the legal capacity to (1) enter into a valid contract? (2) make a will? (3) obtain a marriage license? (4) operate a motor vehicle? (5) vote? or (6) be held civilly liable for his acts in a court of law?

Capacity to Contract

The appointment of a guardian for the person or estate of a mentally retarded individual is an adjudication of his legal incompetency. The effect of this determination on the capacity of the ward to enter into a valid contract is defined in Section 40 of the Civil Code:

> After his incapacity has been judicially determined, a person of unsound mind can make no conveyance or other contract, nor delegate any power or waive any right, until his restoration to capacity.

As interpreted by California case law, Section 40 renders all contracts by mentally retarded wards void:

> When, however, a court has regularly adjudged one to be incompetent, he thereby becomes incapable of making a valid contract, and it is deemed to be void. It seems evident that the term incompetent is intended to include not only the insane, but also those who are afflicted with less serious derangements of the mind. The adjudication of mental incapacity therefore applies to both the insane and the incompetent, regardless of the character or degree of mental derangement.—*Gibson v. Westoby*, 251 P. 2d 1003, 115 C.A. 2d 273 (1953).

A void contract can pass no legal title nor be upheld as legally enforceable in a court of law. The mentally retarded ward, therefore, cannot legally enforce his purchase of a television set, a pair of pants, groceries, etc., or any other commercial agreement.

Most states are not so strict and permit the judicial enforcement of contracts entered into by the ward unless one party to the contract challenges its validity. In these states the contract is characterized as voidable, not void. To the extent that the contract of purchase is for necessaries such as food or essential clothing, many states hold the ward liable for the reasonable value of such goods. The absolute language of Civil Code Section 40, however, rejects both the theory of voidable contracts and liability for necessaries.

Testamentary Capacity

The "testamentary capacity" of a person refers to his ability to make a will. Usually, if a mentally retarded person understands what is involved, he can make a will.

If a mentally retarded person has been placed under a guardianship of his person and/or estate and thereby adjudicated incompetent to enter into a legally enforceable contract, is he also legally incompetent to make a will?

Section 20 of the Probate Code states that "every person of sound mind over the age of 18 years, may dispose of his or her property, real and personal, by will."

In *Johnson's Estate*, 252 P. 1049, 200 Cal. 299 (1927), the court held that an adjudication of incompetency in guardianship proceedings is evidence of the mental condition then existing, but is not prima facie evidence of testamentary incapacity. The fact that a mentally retarded person has been placed under the care of a guardian does *not* conclusively establish his incompetence to make a will. It is only evidence to be weighed with other evidence in the court's attempt to determine if the mentally retarded testator was able to understand the nature and situation of his property and the significance of his planned disposition.

Marriage

Usually, unless a person is severely retarded, he can obtain a marriage license.

Is guardianship conclusive evidence of the ward's inability to obtain a marriage license?

Section 4201 of the California Civil Code lists the persons who are excluded from obtaining a marriage license:

> No license shall be granted when either of the parties, applicants therefore, is an imbecile, or insane, or is at the time of making application for the license, under the influence of any intoxicating liquor, or narcotic drug.

The term "imbecile" is nowhere defined in the California Civil Code or applicable case law. In *Estate of Gregorson*, 160 Cal. 21 (1911), the California Supreme Court indicated that the marriage contract is valid when both parties to the contract possess the requisite mental capacity to consent to marriage. There is no further explanation of what degree of mental impairment prohibits rational consent.

In practice, county clerks in issuing marriage licenses interpret the above statute and case law very liberally. If an applicant demonstrates no aberrational behavior, can speak coherently, and is able to fill out the application in a readable manner, he can obtain a marriage license. Only where the county clerk, on the basis of his initial observations, suspects that the applicant may be so mentally impaired that he cannot rationally consent to marriage will the issue of legal capacity to marry be raised.

Guardianship does *not* conclusively establish mental impairment so that a marriage license cannot be obtained.

In *Hsu v. Mt. Zion Hospital,* 66 Cal. Rptr. 659 (1968), the court indicated that in guardianship cases the presumption of incompetency is applied only to contracts and conveyances and not to wills, marriage, or other "legal acts."

Obtaining a License to Operate a Motor Vehicle

Although the wording in the vehicle code is obsolete in regard to the mentally retarded, most mildly retarded people and some moderately retarded people can obtain driver's licenses.

Section 12805 of the Vehicle Code states that:

> The department shall not issue or renew a driver's license to any person
>
> . . . .
>
> (c) who is insane or feebleminded or an idiot or an imbecile,
> (d) who is an epileptic,
> (e) who is unable as shown by examination to understand traffic signs or signals or does not have a reasonable knowledge of the provisions of this code governing the operations of vehicles upon the highways,
>
> . . . .
>
> (g) Any physical or mental defect of the applicant which in the opinion of the department does not affect the applicant's ability to exercise reasonable and ordinary control in operating a motor vehicle upon the highway shall not prevent the issuance of a license to the applicant.

Though there is no definition of the terms "imbecile," "idiot," or "feebleminded," in the Vehicle Code, if the mentally retarded applicant is able to pass the examination as required by section 12805 (e), he can obtain a driver's license. If the applicant is able to read simple English as required by Subsection (g) but has difficulty reading the written examination, he may take the test orally.

Obtaining a driver's license may be characterized as a "legal act," as that phrase is used in the *Hsu* decision discussed above. Because that opinion states that in guardianship cases the presumption of incompetency is applied only to contracts and conveyances and not to wills, marriage or other "legal acts," the fact that the retarded applicant is under the care of a guardian does not conclusively prevent him from taking the examination and obtaining a license.

Voting

Although it depends somewhat upon the deputy registrar of voters, most mildly and moderately retarded people can become registered voters.

Article 2, Section 1 of the California constitution provides that no idiot or insane person shall exercise the privileges of an elector. The term "idiot" is nowhere defined in the California Election Code, other statutory law of this state or California case law. The insanity exception is embellished in Section 383 of the Election Code:

> The county clerk shall cancel the registration in the following cases:
> ....
> (b) When the insanity of the person registered is legally established.

No further definition of the term "insanity" is provided, nor is it clear what the phrase "legally established" means. Because Article 2, Section 1 of the California constitution recognizes mental deficiency ("idiot") as an impairment separate from mental illness ("insane"), it is doubtful that the term "insanity" on 383 (b) of the Election Code includes the mentally retarded. If the Legislature had intended Section 383 to apply to the mentally retarded, the term "idiot" would have been included.

In an effort to clarify the ambiguity of Section 383 (b), the State Legislature enacted Section 388:

> Every judge before whom proceedings are had which result in any person being declared incapable of managing or taking care of either himself or property or both, and for whom a guardian of his person or estate or both is accordingly appointed, or which result in his being committed to a state hospital as a mentally ill person, shall file with the county clerk a certificate of that fact, and thereupon the county clerk shall cancel the affidavit of registration of that person.

Section 388 made it very clear that the mentally retarded ward under guardianship could not vote in California.

In 1969 Section 388 was repealed. We are once again thrown back to Section 383 (b) which, as was shown above, only refers to the mentally ill or insane. It therefore appears that the mentally retarded person, whether he is under the care of a guardian or not, can vote in California. The only exclusion is found in Article 2, Section 1's undefined, inept and archaic term "idiot." Popular opinion and most dictionary definitions equate "idiot" with the profoundly retarded individual, unable to care for himself and requiring constant supervision. If the applicant is able to understand directions in filling out the affidavit of registration and enter his name and address, he can qualify as a voter.

Eligibility determinations in practice parallel very closely the legal conclusions above. The registrar of voters for the county of San Francisco and the registrar of voters for the county of Sacramento indicated that the decision of whether a person may vote is made by the person who asks the questions and fills in the blank spaces on the affidavit of registration of the prospective voter. If a person is intelligent enough to answer such questions as his name, address, date and place of birth, occupation, and party affiliation, he will be added to the rolls of registered voters by the county clerk. Though the California constitution requires that the applicant be able to read the constitution, no literacy test is given.

Civil Liability

If a retarded person understands what illegal act he has committed and what penalty may be meted out by the court, he is liable for his misdeeds.

Section 41 of the Civil Code states the California rule:

> A minor, or person of unsound mind, of whatever degree, is civilly liable for a wrong done by him, but is not liable in exemplary damages unless at the time of the act he was capable of knowing that it was wrongful.

There is no case law in California dealing specifically with the civil liability of the mentally retarded person. In *Mullen v. Bruce*, 335 P. 2d 945, 168, C.A. 2d 494 (1959), the court observed that Section 41 is a restatement of the common law with respect to the civil liability of minors and incompetents. Most commentators agree that to be held liable for his tortious conduct a person must understand the probable result of his actions. It is not necessary that the actor appreciate the wrongful character of his act, though in some jurisdictions he must desire that the obvious consequence of his act occur. To be found liable for the intentional tort of battery, therefore, the mentally retarded defendant must have understood at the time he committed the tortious act that his conduct would produce a harmful or offensive touching of the plaintiff and in some jurisdictions, he must intend that the harmful result occur.

Guardianship has no effect on the determination of civil liability. In *Campbell v. Bradbury*, 176 P. 685, 179 Cal. 364 (1919), the defendant had been declared incompetent to manage his affairs and a guardian of his estate had been appointed. The plaintiff alleged that the defendant negligently supervised and controlled a building in which an elevator fell injuring the plaintiff. The court held:

> If an insane person, the owner and manager of a business building, would be responsible for the negligent operation of an elevator, notwithstanding his insanity and incapacity, there seems no good reason for holding that he should be exempt therefrom because of the fact that his property was being operated for him by an agent appointed by the court.

Though this case involved an insane defendant, the effect of the defendant's guardianship on civil liability would have been the same had he been mentally retarded.

An adjudication of incompetence resulting from the appointment of a guardian for the person and/or estate of a mentally retarded person means only that the retarded ward is legally incompetent to enter into an enforceable contract. The conclusive presumption of legal incapacity extends no further. The mentally retarded ward may make a will, marry, drive a car, vote and be held civilly liable for his conduct if he meets the appropriate legal requirements.

It is essential that lawyers, parents, social workers and others concerned with the problems of the mentally retarded be aware of the limited legal disabilities which accompany an adjudication of incompetency in guardianship proceedings. If an individual is otherwise qualified to assume the responsibilities of American citizenship, the gloss of incompetence incorrectly associated with guardianship must not prevent him from doing so. Misinterpretation and ignorance of the law should not obstruct the mentally retarded in their effort to become productive members of our society.

Being "normal" in our society is having an I.Q. of 100 so that
You can go to college and get a degree . . .

Being "normal" is being able to walk and run without crutches so
That you can run faster than anyone else and win the race . . .

Being "normal" is having arms and legs like everyone else, so that
You can drive a car . . .

Being "normal" is having the ability to see and hear so that you
Can judge others on their appearance, race or origin . . .

Being "normal" is earning an income so that you can show others
how
Successful you are . . .

But why has man so readily dismissed the essence of every human
being
In his judgment of what is "normal"? His ability to feel—

Love and tenderness have been cast aside too long. . .
And without them, man is simply a machine—performing daily the

Actions of life, yet he is said to be "normal," unfeeling—devoid
Of what makes man "human" . . .

Society judges a man by his outermost possessions more than his
Innermost qualities—a sad mistake by society, but the time
                    For a change is now.

—Christine Koch

Glossary

abscess, brain
: An area of pus formed by the disintegration of brain tissue due to an infection.

acrocephaly
: A malformation in which the head is somewhat pointed because of premature closure of the sutures of the skull.

achondroplasia
: A congenital disease of bone development resulting in dwarfism.

acquired
: Not congenital but occurring after birth.

adenoma
: A benign tumor of glandular origin.

age, mental   Level of intellectual ability in comparison with the average of a particular chronological age group, usually as reflected in intelligence test scores.

albino   A congenital defect (inherited) resulting in a lack of pigmentation of the skin, hair and eyes. No known therapy.

Apert's Syndrome   A condition in which the patient has fused fingers, fused toes, cleft palate, coronal synostosis. Mental retardation results if synostosis is not treated surgically.

alpha rhythm   Normal rhythm seen in adult electroencephalogram varying 8 to 12 cycles per second in frequency.

amaurotic family idiocy   A term no longer used. (See Tay-Sachs Disease.)

amino acids   Any one of a large group of organic compounds which make up proteins. From amino acids the body resynthesizes proteins.

aminoaciduria   Refers to amino acids in urine. An abnormal condition often associated with mental retardation.

amniocentesis   A procedure by which amniotic fluid containing fetal cells is obtained by needle puncture of the pregnant uterus. Cells are then examined microscopically for abnormalities.

amniotic fluid   Fluid surrounding fetus in utero.

anemia   A deficiency in the hemoglobin concentration of the blood, resulting in

	a deficiency in its oxygen-carrying capacity.
anencephaly	Absence of all or part of the brain.
angiomatosis	A congenital vascular defect of the facial skin, producing a large, red discoloration on one side. Usually associated with brain abnormality on the same side as the lesion. Also called Sturge-Weber Syndrome. No therapy available.
anomaly	Abnormality.
anosmia	Absence of the sense of smell.
anoxia	Inadequate supply of oxygen to the brain. Can cause mental retardation if prolonged.
antibiotic	An agent such as penicillin, strep-tomycin, etc., derived from plant life and used to treat infections.
antibody	A substance produced in the blood as a reaction against foreign substances introduced into the bloodstream.
anticonvulsants	Drugs used to control seizures. Supervision by a physician is essential when prescribed.
aphasia	Inability to understand and/or use language meaningfully. This condition may be associated with brain damage.
apnea	A temporary suspension of respiratory exchange of air.
arachnodactyly	Elongated fingers and/or toes. May be associated with Marfan's Syndrome.

arrhythmia

Abnormality of electroencephalogram. Can indicate a tendency toward seizures.

arthrogryposis

Persistent flexure or contracture of joints, inherited in a familial pattern. Occasionally associated with mental retardation. No treatment available.

asphyxia

Suffocation.

astigmatism

A defective formation of those curved surfaces of the eye which reflect light. A hazy image is produced. Correctable with glasses.

ataxia

Impairment of muscular coordination characterized by lack of balance.

athetosis

Involuntary, slow writhing movements, principally of hands and feet, due to a brain lesion. Treatment with physical therapy.

atrophy

Wasting away or diminution in size of a tissue, organ or part.

audiogram

A graph of the variations of the acuteness of hearing of an individual.

aura

A peculiar sensation that precedes an epileptic attack.

autism

A disorder in which the person does not respond normally to stimulation and seems to act in response to internal demands. He is often said to "live in a world of his own." May be associated with brain damage, convulsions, or prematurity. Can be treated by attendance at day-care programs and by drugs, depending on symptoms. Results of treatment vary.

autosome
An ordinary chromosome as distinguished from a sex-determining chromosome.

Babinski reflex test
An abnormal reaction elicited by stroking or stimulating the sole of the foot. With a positive Babinski reaction, the toes extend (especially the big toe) and spread. It occurs in lesions of the motor tracts in the central nervous system.

benign
Not malignant. Favorable for recovery.

bilirubin
A bile pigment. Excessive amounts in the blood and tissues can cause brain damage due to decreased oxygen uptake.

borderline
The level of intellectual ability between mental retardation and normal. IQ level is usually 70–85.

brachial palsy
Paralysis or partial paralysis of the arm resulting from injury to the nerves at birth.

brain injury
A general term which refers to any damage to the brain.

cataract
Opacity of the crystalline lens of the eye. Can be removed surgically.

central nervous system
All parts of the brain and spinal cord.

cephalic delivery
Normal, head-first delivery of a baby.

cerebellum	The lower part of the brain involved in muscle coordination and maintenance of bodily equilibrium.
cerebral angiogram	A radiograph of the brain made visible by injection of radiopaque dye into the cerebral arteries.
cerebral palsy	Neuromuscular dysfunction due to brain damage.
cerebrospinal	Pertaining to the brain and the spinal cord.
cerebrum	The upper right and left region of the brain.
cervical	Pertaining to the neck.
chorea	A nervous disorder characterized by involuntary, jerking movements of extremities and facial muscles. Usually occurs secondary to a streptococcal infection. Not associated with mental retardation.
chromosome	The structures in the cell nucleus which carry the genes (hereditary factors). Humans normally have 46 chromosomes in each cell.
chromosomal abnormality	Refers to a numerical abnormality such as a monosomy, trisomy or mosaicism. Also a structural abnormality such as a deletion, translocation or inversion of a chromosome.
chronic	Not acute. Prolonged.
cirrhosis	Inflammatory disease of the liver resulting in the development of excess fibrous tissue within that organ.

cleft palate	A congenital defect due to a failure in development of the roof of the mouth. Repaired surgically.
clonic movements	Abnormal repetitive movements of the foot. May be induced by a sudden pushing up of the foot while the leg is extended. If present after 4 or 5 months of age, it indicates neurological damage.
coma	A state of complete loss of consciousness from which the patient cannot be aroused even by powerful stimulation.
concussion	Reaction of the brain due to a blow upon the head attended by dizziness, nausea, loss of consciousness, weak pulse, and slow respiration.
congenital	Present at birth.
contusion	A bruise which does not break the skin.
convulsive disorder	Convulsions; epilepsy; seizures; fits. A condition caused by brain dysfunction and resulting in abnormal involuntary movements of the body. Preventive therapy with drugs.
cornea	Front transparent part of the external layer of the eyeball.
Cornelia de Lange Syndrome	A condition in which the patient has skeletal deformities, deafness, heavy arched eyebrows and usually severe mental retardation.
cortex	The outer substance of an organ as distinguished from its inner substance. The cerebral cortex is the

	portion of the brain having to do with reasoning.
coxsackie	Virus infection. Usually respiratory.
craniopharyngioma	An intracranial tumor arising from the craniopharyngeal duct in the area of the pituitary gland. Surgical treatment is effective if done early.
craniosynostosis	Premature closure of the cranial sutures. Can be repaired surgically. Mental retardation can be prevented if the operation is done early.
cranium	The skull.
Crouzon's Disease	Ocular hypertelorism (widely spaced eyes). Hereditary disease sometimes associated with mental retardation.
cyanosis	Blueness of the mucous membranes and sometimes of the skin due to insufficient oxygen in the blood.
cytomegalic disease	Virus infection of the mother causing defects in the fetus. No proven treatment at present.
degeneration	Deterioration.
developmental quotient	Score obtained from a developmental test during infancy to determine the level of functioning.
diagnosis	Identification of a disease.
diplegia	Paralysis affecting like parts on both sides of the body, such as both arms or both legs.
diplopia	The seeing of single objects as double. Double vision.
dorsal	Pertaining to the back or upper part.

dull-normal	A term sometimes used to describe the intelligence of individuals obtaining IQ scores from 70 to 85. Slow learner.
dura	Tough, fibrous covering of the brain.
dysplasia	Developmental abnormality or failure to develop normally. Some disorders cause dysplasia of the tooth enamel.
educable retarded	Refers to those persons who are able to learn elementary school skills, such as reading, writing and arithmetic. The IQ range of this group is roughly between 50 and 70.
electroencephalogram	The record produced by an electroencephalograph, an instrument used to record changes in electric potential between different areas of the brain.
encephalitis	Inflammation of the brain, usually due to a virus.
endocrine	Pertaining to those glands whose secretions pass directly into the bloodstream.
enuresis	Bed wetting.
epicanthal folds	Vertical folds of skin at the inner corners of the eyes. A symptom of Down's syndrome.
epilepsy	See convulsive disorders.
erythroblastosis	A condition characterized by anemia, jaundice and enlarged liver and spleen due to Rh incompatibility.

familial	Tendency to occur among members of an affected family.
feeble-mindedness	A term occasionally used as a synonym for mental retardation, but no longer used by professionals.
fetus	The unborn offspring, principally from the end of the third month to birth.
flaccid	Lack of tone. Weakness.
fontanel	The space between the cranial bones covered by a membranous structure. Soft spot present at the top of a normal infant's head at birth.
galactosemia	An inborn error of metabolism producing a defect or deficiency in the enzyme which converts galactose to glucose. Detectable by blood test. If untreated, causes mental retardation. Treatable with diet. Mental retardation can be prevented if treatment is started early.
gamete	An egg or sperm.
ganglion	A collection of nerve cells that serves as a center of nerve control.
gargoylism	One of a group of diseases due to an enzyme defect involving many body tissues. Characterized by dwarf stature, shortness of neck and trunk, depression of the bridge of the nose, clouding of the corneas of the eyes. No treatment. Preventable only by prenatal diagnosis.
gene	Those parts of the chromosome which transmit hereditary characteristics.

genetic	Pertaining to or transmitted by genes.
gestation	Length of pregnancy.
gland	An organ that produces a secretion.
glaucoma	An insidious eye disease caused by difficulty in the circulation of the fluid substance of the eyeball; this condition results in abnormal pressure within the eyeball. Blindness often results if treatment is delayed.
glycogen	A carbohydrate substance found in abundance in the liver and muscles.
grand mal seizure	A major seizure preceded by an aura. A sharp onset with tonic and clonic movements and loss of consciousness. Most seizures can be controlled with drugs.
hematoma	Tissue swelling containing blood.
hemiparesis	Slight paralysis of the muscles of one side of the body. Physical therapy treatment.
hemiplegia	Paralysis of one side of the body. Physical therapy treatment.
heterozygote	A carrier of a genetic defect.
histidinemia	An enzyme defect of histidine metabolism sometimes associated with mental retardation. Treatable by diet.
homocystinuria	An enzyme defect in methionine (an amino acid) metabolism. Associated with mental retardation. Treatable with diet and vitamin B_6 therapy.

homozygous	Pertaining to members of a pair of genes which are alike with respect to the characteristics represented.
Hurler's Disease	See gargoylism.
hydrocephalus	Head enlargement due to abnormal increase in the amount of cerebrospinal fluid and accompanied by dilation of the cerebral ventricles. This disorder can usually be prevented by surgical intervention.
hyperactivity	Excessive and uncontrollable movement, such as is found in persons with central nervous system damage. Also anxiety. Controllable with drugs or environmental change.
hyperbilirubinemia	Excessive amount of bilirubin in the blood, such as occurs in cases of blood Rh incompatibility. Treatment: exchange transfusion or photo therapy.
hypertelorism	Widely spaced eyes.
hyperopia	Farsightedness; the lack of refracting power sufficient to focus the light rays reflected from objects close to the eyes. Treatable with glasses.
hyperglycinemia	Amino acid disorder of metabolism associated with mental retardation. Treatable by diet.
hypoglycemia	Deficiency of blood sugar. Treatment with diet or hormones, depending on the cause.
hypoplasia, cerebral	Underdevelopment of brain tissue.

hypothyroidism — Underfunctioning of the thyroid gland. Diagnosed through blood and bone studies. Treatable with oral administration of thyroid hormone. Mental retardation can be prevented if treatment is started early.

hypotonia — Reduction in muscle tone. Treated by physical therapy.

hypsarrhythmia — Unusual electroencephalographic pattern of myoclonic seizures.

idiopathic — Pertaining to spontaneous or unknown origin of a disease.

inflammation — A tissue reaction manifested by redness and swelling.

intelligence test — A procedure in which mental age is measured.

intelligence quotient — Ratio of mental age to chronological age multiplied by 100.

intoxication — A poisoning.

in utero — Within the uterus.

jaundice — A condition characterized by yellowish skin due to the presence of excess bile pigments (bilirubin) in the tissues and bloodstream.

kernicterus — Damage to certain collections of cells in the brain due to high bilirubin levels in the blood and tissues.

kwashiorkor — A condition due to protein deficiency characterized by fatty infiltration of liver and pigmentary changes of the skin. Associated with chronic malnutrition.

lesion

A localized structural change or abnormality.

leucine-sensitive
hypoglycemia

Unusual form of low blood sugar syndrome induced by the amino acid leucine. Causes mental retardation. Treatable with diet low in leucine.

Lowe's Syndrome

See oculo-cerebral-renal syndrome. No treatment.

malnutrition

Grossly inadequate nutrition.

maple syrup urine disease

Rare disorder of amino acid metabolism, characterized by convulsions and mental retardation. Dietary treatment prevents mental retardation.

Marfan's Syndrome

A condition in which the patient has congenital heart disease, elongated fingers and toes, and has cataracts. No treatment.

meiosis

A process occurring in the formation of gametes in which the number of chromosomes is reduced by half.

mental subnormality

A general term to describe the mentally retarded. This term is used in the United Kingdom.

metabolism

Process of producing, maintaining and destroying body tissues.

metaphase

The second stage of mitosis in which the chromosomes split.

methylmalonicaciduria

Defect in metabolism of methylmalonic acid (product of protein metabolism). Causes mental retardation. Treatable with diet and B_{12}.

microcephaly	An abnormally small cranium. A characteristic of some forms of mental retardation.
mitosis	Reproduction of cells.
Mongolism	Obsolete term denoting Down's syndrome. A chromosomal condition in which the individual has certain physical characteristics, and is almost always mentally retarded to one degree or another.
Moro reflex	On sudden removal of support, an infant cries and throws his arms outward and then brings them together; the fingers are extended at first and then the hands are closed. Also called startle reflex.
mosaicism	A condition in which an individual has an abnormal number of chromosomes in some cells and a normal chromosomal complement in other cells.
myoclonic seizures	A form of epileptic seizure in which the patient repeatedly drops the head and extends the arms.
myopia	Near-sightedness. Correctable with glasses.
myotonia	Increased muscle tone due to disease of the nervous system.
neonatal	Pertaining to the period of time between onset of labor and six weeks of age.
neuritis	Inflammation of a nerve with pain and tenderness. Underlying cause must be treated.

neurologist	A physician trained in the treatment of diseases of the nervous system.
neurosurgery	Surgery of the nervous system.
nystagmus	Involuntary rapid movement of the eyeball.
oculo-cerebral-renal syndrome (Lowe's Syndrome)	Rare sex-linked disorder of amino acid metabolism characterized by cataracts, mental retardation, hypotonia and aminoaciduria.
ophthalmologist	A physician who specializes in the eye and diseases of the eye.
optic atrophy	Degeneration of the optic nerve manifested by pallor of the optic disc.
palsy, cerebral	Term used to denote impairment of motor function due to a brain lesion.
paralysis	Loss or impairment of motor function in a part due to lesion of the neural or muscular mechanism.
paraplegia	Paralysis of the legs and lower part of the body.
perception	The receiving of an impression through the senses.
petit mal epilepsy	A mild attack of epilepsy characterized by a transient loss of consciousness. Controlled by drugs.
phenylalanine	An amino acid essential in human nutrition.
phenylketonuria	A disease due to a defect or absence of an enzyme which facilitates the conversion of phenylalanine to tyrosine. Dietary treatment available. Causes mental retardation if not treated.

photo therapy	The use of fluorescent lights to reduce jaundice.
pneumoencephalogram	X-ray of the brain after injection of the ventricles with air or gas via the spinal cord. Used for diagnostic purposes.
postmature	This term refers to a condition in which the fetus is delivered following a gestation period greater than forty-two weeks.
postnatal	After birth.
premature	A baby born before the expected date and requiring special attention because of the immaturity of his body functions. A baby who weighs less than 5 pounds 8 ounces at birth.
prenatal	Before birth.
prognosis	Forecast of the course and outcome of a disease.
prosthesis	An artificial part, such as a limb, eye or denture.
protozoa	A subdivision (phylum) of the animal kingdom made up of organisms consisting of a single cell.
psychosis	A disorder of behavior characterized by loss of contact with reality.
quadriplegia	Motor dysfunction of all four extremities.
Rh factor	A blood factor which may cause blood transfusion reactions.
reflex	An automatic action or motion often elicited by tapping the muscle tendon.

retrolental fibroplasia	Fibrous overgrowth of vascular tissue in the eye, occurring in premature infants because of excessive administration of oxygen. Causes blindness.
rigidity	Muscular immobility.
roentgenogram	An X-ray photograph.
rubella	German measles or three-day measles.
sagittal	Midline. Sagittal suture refers to the midline suture of the skull.
scaphocephaly	A condition in which the skull presents a boat-shaped appearance due to premature ossification of the sagittal suture. Treatment by neurosurgery.
sclerosis	Induration or hardening.
spasticity	Increasing tone of the muscles, making it difficult for the person to control the extremities. Treatment by physical therapy.
spina bifida	A congenital malformation consisting of a defect in the vertebrae through which the contents of the spinal canal may protrude. Treatment is available depending upon severity of the condition. Often causes mental retardation.
strabismus	Cross-eye; a visual defect characterized by inability to direct the eyes to the same point as a result of incoordination of ocular muscles. Correctable through surgery or glasses.

subdural hematoma	A blood clot beneath the dura of the brain usually due to injury. Treatment: neurosurgery.
symptom	Any evidence of disease or of a patient's condition.
syndrome	A specific collection of symptoms.
Tay-Sachs Disease	A fatal, hereditary, recessive disease occurring almost exclusively in children of Ashkenazi Jewish descent. Symptoms are usually manifested by the fourth month of life. Characterized by convulsions, spasticity and progressive blindness marked by the appearance of a cherry-red spot in the retina of the eye associated with optic atrophy. No treatment. Preventable by amniocentesis.
thrombosis	The formation of a clot in the blood vessel or in one of the cavities of the heart. Caused by coagulation of the blood.
thyroid	A gland in the neck near the larynx, containing an organic iodine compound, thyroxin. Congenital absence of the thyroid causes cretinism, a form of dwarfism with mental retardation.
tonic movement	Increased muscle tension.
toxemia	A condition in which the blood contains toxic or poisonous substances.
toxoplasmosis	Infection with a genus of protozoan organisms which is transmitted to the baby before birth from the mother.

trisomic — Three chromosomes instead of two.

tuberous sclerosis — A familial disease characterized by mental retardation, convulsions, skin changes and occasional brain tumors. Untreatable.

tyrosine — An amino acid found in protein substances.

ventricle — Any small cavity, especially either one of the two lower (right and left) cavities of the heart or any one of the several cavities of the brain.

ventriculogram — X-ray of the brain after injection of air into the cerebral ventricles directly through the brain by needle.

WBC — Abbreviation for white blood count.

Warkany's Syndrome — Congenital disorder characterized by dwarfism, prominent nose, microcephaly and mental retardation.

Wilson's Disease — Disease caused by abnormal copper deposits in many organs of the body. Drug treatment now available.

X-chromosome — Sex-determining chromosome. In most species, females have two X-chromosomes.

Y-chromosome — Sex-determining chromosome. Males have one Y-chromosome paired with one X-chromosome.

Bibliography

BLATT, BURTON. *Exodus from Pandemonium*. Boston: Allyn and Bacon, Inc., 1970.

BRAZELTON, T. BERRY. *Infants and Mothers*. New York: Dell Publishing Co., Inc., 1972.

BUCK, PEARL. *The Child Who Never Grew*. New York: The John Day Co., 1950.

CARTER, C. O. *Human Heredity*. Baltimore, Md.: Penguin Books, Inc., 1962.

CAUGHEY, JOHN. *To Kill a Child's Spirit*. Itasca, Ill. F. E. Peacock Publishers, Inc., 1973.

CHIGIER, E. *Downs Syndrome*. Lexington, Mass.: Lexington Books, 1973.

COLEMAN, JAMES C. *Abnormal Psychology and Modern Life*. Chicago: Scott, Foresman and Company, 1966.

CRUICKSHANK, WILLIAM M. *The Teacher of Brain-Injured Children*. Syracuse, N.Y.: Syracuse University Press, 1966.

DORFMAN, ALBERT. *Antenatal Diagnosis*. Chicago: The University of Chicago Press, 1972.

287

DYBWAD, GUNNAR. *Challenges in Mental Retardation.* New York and London: Columbia University Press, 1964.

EVANS, DALE. *Angel Unaware.* Westwood, N.J.: Revell Publishing Co., 1953.

EGG, MARIA. *When a Child Is Different.* New York: The John Day Co., 1964.

———. *Educating the Child Who Is Different.* New York: The John Day Co., 1964.

———. *The Different Child Grows Up.* New York: The John Day Co., 1969.

ENNIS, BRUCE J., and PAUL R. FRIEDMAN, with the assistance of BONNIE GITLIN (eds.), *Legal Rights of the Mentally Handicapped,* 3 vols. New York: Practicing Law Institute, 1973.

FINNIE, NANCIE R. *Handling the Young Cerebral Palsied Child at Home.* London: Spottswood, Ballantyne and Co., Ltd., 1968.

GORDON, SOL. *Facts About Sex.* New York: The John Day Co., 1969.

JOHNSON, ERIC W. *Love and Sex in Plain Language.* Philadelphia and New York: J. B. Lippincott, 1967.

KING, MARTIN LUTHER, JR. *Where Do We Go from Here: Chaos or Community?* New York: Harper & Row, Publishers, Inc., 1968.

KOCH, RICHARD, and JAMES C. DOBSON. *The Mentally Retarded Child and His Family.* New York: Brunner/Mazel, Publishers, 1971.

NURNBERGER, JOHN I. (ed.). *Biological and Environmental Determinants of Early Development.* Baltimore, Md.: The Williams and Wilkens Co., 1973.

Report of the National Advisory Commission on Civil Disorders. New York: Bantam Books, Inc., 1968.

ROSENTHAL, ROBERT, and LENORE JACOBSON. *Pygmalion in the Classroom.* New York: Holt, Rinehart and Winston, Inc., 1969.

SKEELS, H. M. "Effects of Adoption on Children from Institutions," *Children,* Vol. 12 (1965).

———, and E. A. FILLMORE. "The Mental Development of Children from Underprivileged Homes," *Journal of Genetic Psychology,* Vol. 50 (1937).

SMITH, DAVID W., and ANN A. WILSON. *The Child with Downs Syndrome.* Philadelphia: Saunders Co., 1973.

THOMPSON, TRAVIS, and JOHN GRABOWSKI. *Behavior Modification of the Mentally Retarded.* New York and London: Oxford University Press, 1972.

Helpful Organizations and Publications

American Association for Mental Deficiency
5201 Connecticut Ave., N.W.
Washington, D.C., 20015

Atypical Infant Development Program (kit available for new
  parents)
1030 Sir Francis Drive
Kentfield, Cal.

California Tay-Sachs Disease Prevention Program
Harbor General Hospital
1000 W. Carson Street, E4
Torrance, Cal. 90509

The Canadian Association for the Mentally Retarded
York University Campus
4700 Keele St.
Downsville (Toronto), Ontario, Canada M3 J 1P3

Downs Syndrome Congress (monthly newsletter)
1800 Rhodesia Ave.
Friendly, Md. 20022

Epilepsy Foundation of America
1828 L St., N.W., Suite 406
Washington, D.C., 20036

Handicapped Children's Education Project
A project of the Education Commission of the States (46 states
 and territories)
300 Lincoln Tower, 1860 Lincoln St.
Denver, Colo. 80203

International League of Societies for the Mentally Handicapped
12 Forestière
Brussels, Belgium

Liaison (published monthly, reporting programs and citizen involvement in serving the developmentally disabled)
744 P St., Suite 724
Sacramento, Cal. 95814

Mental Health Law Project
1751 N St., N.W.
Washington, D.C., 20036

Mental Retardation and the Law (monthly publication)
U.S. Department of Health, Education and Welfare
Office of the Assistant for Human Development
Office of Mental Retardation Coordination
Washington, D.C., 20201

Mothers of Young Mongoloids
713 Ramsey St.
Alexandria, Va. 22301

National Association for Downs Syndrome
628 Ashland
Chicago, Ill. 60305

National Association for Retarded Citizens (NARC)
2709 Ave. E East, P.O. Box 6109
Arlington, Texas 76011

The following list of individual state offices of the Association for Retarded Citizens (ARC) has been provided to us courtesy of this organization. Any state office can provide information on local ARC groups within the state.

Alabama ARC
2125 E. South Blvd.
Montgomery, Ala. 36111

Alaska ARC
3331 Tudor Rd.
Anchorage, Alas. 99502

Arizona ARC
2929 E. Thomas Rd., Rm. 216
Phoenix, Ariz. 85016

Arkansas ARC
University Shopping Center, Asher at University
Little Rock, Ark. 72204

California ARC
1225 Eighth St., Suite 312
Sacramento, Cal. 95814

Colorado ARC
634 S. Broadway
Denver, Col. 80209

Connecticut ARC, Inc.
21-R High St.
Hartford, Conn. 06103

Delaware ARC, Inc.
P.O. Box 1896
Wilmington, Del. 19899

District of Columbia ARC
405 Riggs Rd., N.E.
Washington, D.C., 20001

Florida ARC, Inc.
P.O. Box 1542
Tallahassee, Fla. 32302

Georgia ARC, Inc.
1575 Phoenix Blvd., Suite 8
Atlanta, Ga. 30349

Hawaii ARC
245 Kukui St.
Honolulu, Hawaii 96807

Idaho ARC
P.O. Box 816, 430 N. 9th St.
Boise, Id. 83701

Illinois ARC
343 S. Dearborn St., Rm. 709
Chicago, Ill. 60604

Indiana ARC
752 E. Market St.
Indianapolis, Ind. 46202

Iowa ARC, Inc.
1707 High St.
Des Moines, Ia. 50309

Kansas ARC, Inc.
6100 Martway, Suite 1
Mission, Kans. 66202

Kentucky ARC, Inc.
State Office Building Annex
Frankfort, Ky. 40601

Louisiana ARC
6844 Van Gogh Dr.
Baton Rouge, La. 70806

Maine ARC
269 ½ Water St.
Augusta, Me. 04330

Maryland ARC
20 Gwynns Mill Court
Owings Mills, Md. 21117

Massachusetts ARC, Inc.
381 Elliot St.
Newton Upper Falls, Mass. 02164

Michigan ARC
510 National Tower Bldg.
Lansing, Mich. 48933

Minnesota ARC
3225 Lyndale Ave.
Minneapolis, Minn. 55408

Missouri ARC
Box 1363, 145 E. Amite
Jefferson City, Mo. 65101

Montana ARC, Inc.
P.O. Box 625
Helena, Mont. 59601

Nebraska ARC
140 South 27
Lincoln, Neb. 69510

Nevada ARC, Inc.
1125 Cashman Dr.
Las Vegas, Nev. 89102

New Hampshire ARC
4 Park St.
Concord, N.H. 03301

New Jersey ARC
99 Bayard St.
New Brunswick, N.J. 08901

New Mexico ARC
8200 ½ Menaul Blvd., N.E., Suite 3
Albuquerque, N.M. 87110

North Carolina ARC, Inc.
P.O. Box 18551
Raleigh, N.C. 27609

North Dakota ARC, Inc.
514 ½ 1st Ave. N, P.O. Box 1494
Fargo, N.D. 58102

Ohio ARC
61 E. Gay St.
Columbus, Ohio 43215

Oklahoma ARC
Box 14250
Oklahoma City, Okla. 73114

Oregon ARC
3085 River Road N.,
Salem, Oreg. 97303

Pennsylvania ARC
127 Locust St.
Harrisburg, Pa. 17101

Puerto Rico ARC
GPO Box 1904
San Juan, P.R. 00936

Rhode Island ARC
Snow Building, 2845 Post Rd.
Warwick, R.I. 02886

South Carolina ARC, Inc.
P.O. Box 1564
Columbia, S.C. 29202

South Dakota ARC
111 W. Capitol, P.O. Box 502
Pierre, S.D. 57212

Tennessee ARC, Inc.
2121 Belcourt Ave.
Nashville, Tenn. 37212

Texas ARC
833 W. Houston
Austin, Tex. 78756

Utah ARC, Inc.
2952 South 7th East
Salt Lake City, Utah 84106

Vermont ARC, Inc.
RFD
Bellows Falls, Vt. 05101

Virginia ARC
809 Mutual Building
909 E. Main St.
Richmond, Va. 23219

Washington ARC
213 ½ E. 4th, Suite 10
Olympia, Wash. 98501

West Virginia ARC
Union Trust Bldg., Rm. 614
Parkersburg, W.Va. 26101

Wisconsin ARC, Inc.
351 W. Washington Ave.
Madison, Wis. 53703

Wyoming ARC, Inc.
Box C
Buffalo, Wyo. 82834

Opincar Chapter ARC
Frankfurt Elementary School #1
APO
New York, N.Y. 09757

National Information and Referral Service for Autistic and
Autistic-Like Persons
101 Richmond St.
Huntington, W.Va. 25702

National Society for Autistic Children, Inc.
621 Central Ave.
Albany, N.Y. 12206

Parents Anonymous (90 chapters)
2930 W. Imperial Highway
Inglewood, Cal. 90303

Parents of Mongoloids
1519 Antigua Lane
Houston, Tex. 77058

United Cerebral Palsy Association (National)
66 E. 34th St.
New York City, N.Y.

Index

About the Authors

RICHARD KOCH, who was born in Dickinson, North Dakota, in 1921, was graduated from the University of Rochester School of Medicine and took his specialty training in pediatrics at Childrens Hospital in Los Angeles. He subsequently became director of the Child Development Division at Childrens Hospital, a position he still holds; he is also professor of pediatrics at University of Southern California School of Medicine. He has held numerous committee appointments at the local, state and national levels, and is a former president of the California Association for the Retarded and of the American Association on Mental Deficiency. At present he is a member of the National Research Advisory Board of the National Association for Retarded Citizens. As the director of a regional center serving developmentally disabled persons, Dr. Koch has gained wide experience in dealing with the handicapped and their families. He has published more than eighty articles and is the co-author of *The Mentally Retarded Child and His Family*, published in 1972. In 1974 he received the Distinguished Service Award from Childrens Hospital in recognition of his services to retarded children and adults.

KATHRYN JEAN KOCH is a native Californian, and received her B.A. degree and elementary teaching credential from San Jose State College in 1946. Her special interests have been in the fields of human relations and conservation; she was chairman of the Westchester Human Relations Council for two years and served on the board of directors of the Westside Fair Housing Council. Since 1965 she has been a leader in the battle to protect Mineral King in the Sierras of California from being developed and commercialized; she is secretary of the Mineral King Task Force of the Sierra Club.

Dr. and Mrs. Koch are the parents of three daughters and two sons. The whole family enjoys the outdoors and spends some time skiing each winter and back-packing each summer. They have climbed to the top of Mt. Whitney and back-packed to the bottom of the Grand Canyon.